NURSING YOUR CHILD AT HOME

NURSING YOUR CHILD AT HOME

Supporting Your Child Through Fever Naturally

RACHÆL GOSLING

Matador
9 Priory Business Park,
Wistow Road, Kibworth Beauchamp,
Leicestershire. LE8 0RX
Tel: 0116 279 2299
Email: books@troubador.co.uk
Web: www.troubador.co.uk/matador
Twitter: @matadorbooks

ISBN 978 1788033 152

British Library Cataloguing in Publication Data.
A catalogue record for this book is available from the British Library.

Printed and bound by CPI Group (UK) Ltd, Croydon, CR0 4YY
Typeset in 11pt Aldine 401 BT by Troubador Publishing Ltd, Leicester, UK

Cover design by Alex Segreti

Matador is an imprint of Troubador Publishing Ltd

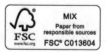

Dedications

To Pete, Claudia and Joshua

To Lori

To all the Mums and Dads up in the small hours with a poorly child

To Coco and Bunker

Fai fai lemu

Disclaimer

The products and companies mentioned and recommended in this book come from the author's own independent experience and use. The author has not benefitted financially or in any other way from the endorsements in this book.

All remedies and advice contained in this book are suggestions only and should not substitute the opinion of a qualified medical professional or health practitioner. Do not attempt to diagnose or self-prescribe for children, especially those with medical complications or who are taking medication.

The information in this book is based on the experiences and research of the author and is not definitive or absolute. Every child is unique and will respond uniquely to care and treatment. The publisher and author are not responsible for any outcomes, consequences or adverse effects that may occur as a result of following the information, instructions and remedies contained in this book.

Wholistic vs Holistic

I know this is going to irritate some of you, but I would like to explain and justify my use of the word wholistic in this book instead of holistic before we begin.

Wholistic conveys both visually and aurally the root of the word whole. For me it beautifully demonstrates the completeness, the all-encompassing nature of the philosophy and theory of nursing care I am advocating throughout this book. The whole child is considered in terms of their physical, emotional and spiritual needs, as well as considering their environmental, nutritional and medical requirements. This book encourages parents and carers to create a picture of every aspect that impacts and governs their child's health both in sickness and on their journey to recovery.

Holistic, in contrast, appears like a dark tunnel, a hole that is empty and full of echoes. It is almost the antithesis of what this book is about, and I felt compelled to resist using it. I apologise if my choice causes confusion or irritation for some of you, but I hope you understand why I favour wholistic over holistic, and that you don't hold it against me!

Thanks and Appreciation

A special thanks to all the amazing doctors and nurses who I have been privileged enough to work with and learn from, especially the Surrey University and Royal Surrey gang! To Jeanette, thank you for showing me another way.

Also, a massive thank you to Jane Gotto for introducing me to the world of complementary therapies, many, many years ago. Thank you to the amazing people at The Beacon and Weleda NZ for letting me work with you and learn from you. A very special thank you goes to all the healers, herbalists, homeopaths and therapists, mainstream and traditional, who I have been fortunate enough to meet all over the world, in the most random and bizarre places sometimes! I have learnt so much from each of you.

Thanks to James, Em, Susie and Alex who have helped edit and design this book. Yes, I needed a team to sort my grammar out! A special thanks goes to Ping, Beccy and all the Bootcamp ladies who are just amazing. Finally, thank you to everyone who has helped distract me over a hot coffee – you know who you are!

Contents

"Watch over us. Wrap us up against the cold and the rain, and give us shade from the hot sun. Make sure we have enough to eat and drink and if we are sick, nurse and comfort us."

Right Number 24

For Every Child
The rights of the child in words and pictures
(UNICEF, 2002)

Based on The United Nations Convention on the Rights of the Child

Preface

This book is written for parents and carers who are looking to take a more proactive role in nursing their child through common childhood illness, and gain a better understanding of the wholistic concepts that support and help to govern child health. The aim is to embrace the well-trodden path of what we now call 'complementary therapies', but which were once the mainstay of healthcare in our communities, and combine this traditional knowledge with the sound medical advice and research that we are privileged to have access to today.

We used to turn to the Wise Women of the community; those with knowledge of herbs and healing, who had vast experience of caring for the children of the village. These wonderful women were a valuable resource of recipes and soothing therapies to comfort the sickening child. A Wise Woman would have known both the child she was ministering to and intricate details about the child's family and social environment. Indeed, she may very well have tended to the birth of that child.

My hope is that this book will help to calm, reassure, advise and give support and solace when it is most needed. To combine the best remedies from a number of complementary fields with conventional medical common sense that is age appropriate. In short, I hope it will act as a portable Wise Woman for treating fever, to build the confidence of the nurse, parent or carer tending to the child.

We appear to have become afraid of sickness and fever, especially in children. We have a growing dependence on pharmaceuticals and those considered "'qualified'" to care for our children. While there is certainly a place for pharmaceuticals and medical professionals, the expert on your child and the health of your child is you. In many instances, there is a lack of confidence in our own ability to care for our children through illness. Children will at times become unwell, and children need to be allowed to be ill. They need to experience common childhood illness fully, not masked or inhibited by our pharmaceutical crutches; they need to allow their miraculous bodies and complex immune systems to kick in and flex their mighty muscles. In allowing this, combined with ensuring good nutrition, ample rest and proper supportive care, we can help our children to become stronger and more resilient. In a world potentially without, or at best with very limited numbers of effective antibiotics, this is exactly where we need to focus our attention.

Initially, it can be quite a terrifying journey for a parent used to dosing a child with medication at the first sign of a fever. It is a mindset that even those in the medical profession struggle with, despite the weight of scientific evidence and even NICE (National Institute of Care Excellence) guidelines stipulating that fever, in and of itself, in a normally healthy child should not be suppressed for the sake of it. There are other ways of making your child feel more comfortable, and I hope to delve into this further in the book. But after just a couple of occasions when a child is allowed to be ill, in most cases the parent or carer will notice that the child appears not as sickly as others, recovers faster and with fewer complications. Once you see this happen, you will grow more confident in your ability to support your child through illness and build their health and resilience.

Frequently the demands of modern life make it difficult to allow the time for children to be ill. With the breakdown of traditional communities and families, combined with the demands financially on a household requiring all adult members to work, who can afford to stay at home and care for a sick child? I am not here to judge, and I hope that even parents who are not able to totally immerse themselves in the philosophy of this book can still take what they need from it. Also, I am aware that some readers will be well versed and qualified in the methods of care suggested within this book, while some readers will have no experience at all. I have written this book from the perspective of someone who is new to caring for a sick child using more natural and observational methods, so some of the suggestions may seem very obvious to more experienced carers, but I hope there will be some useful insights too.

This book is for you to use how and when you please. It should not inhibit or prevent anyone from seeking medical advice and attention for their child. If it is necessary, even just for peace of mind, then you must do it. Always follow your instinct and use your own knowledge and common sense. This book is intended to share information and experiences, not give a definitive diagnosis or guaranteed cure.

I have been lucky enough to have met wonderful people with outstanding knowledge in supporting child health naturally, and the mainstay of their practice is based on simplicity: simple effective treatments given calmly to the child with a nurturing hand. I have seen this principle at play across many cultures, oceans and seas, and I hope this book guides you in the same simple, supportive way, building your confidence, inspiring you to seek further knowledge and bringing empowerment to you within your home to nurse your family.

I wish you all the best and hope that you find something in this book that helps and is of interest to you.

Rachael Gosling
October 2016

How to Use this Book

This book is divided into two parts. Part One is intended to be read as a whole and explains the theories and philosophies that form the basis of this book.

Part Two is intended to be referred to as and when needed. Part Two covers not only the practical hands-on stuff, but is also designed for practicality of use. Suggested treatments and remedies have been divided into age-specific sections and each section is designed to be completely self-contained. For instance, if you have an 18-month-old child then all the appropriate treatments can be found in the section that covers children who are 18 months old. Part Two also contains instructions on practical nursing therapies, recipes and gives some space for you to make your own notes. It is not designed to be read as a whole, but to be dipped in and out of as required, section by section.

The book has been designed like this for clarity and ease of use. There is nothing worse than feeling flustered and exhausted when your child is unwell, flicking backwards and forwards through a book trying to find information like a woman (or man!) possessed! I really hope this layout helps you find what you need quickly, easily and all in one place.

Part One

Chapter One

An Introduction to Fever

A fever (or 'pyrexia' as it is referred to by medical professionals) is defined as a raised body temperature of 37.3 degrees Celsius (98.6 Fahrenheit) or higher. In practice, a fever is not considered significant until it reaches 38 degrees Celsius (100.4 Fahrenheit) or higher.

I need to start this chapter by saying that a young baby, certainly up to three months of age, should always be seen by a medical professional if they get a fever. This is because fever in young babies is quite unusual, as they would normally have protection against infections from their mother's antibodies during this time. Once a doctor's diagnosis has been given, you are free to decide on the course of treatment you prefer for your child. If you are ever worried or concerned about your child then always seek advice from a qualified professional, and ideally one who knows your child and family well, both in times of health and sickness, so they can truly assess the child and support the family appropriately.

Having said that, I need to ask that you change how you view fever. It is likely to go against many things you have been told and many things that you hold to be absolutely and irrefutably true. I need you to try and stop seeing fever as a symptom of the illness and start seeing fever for what it really is; namely the immune system functioning as it should in order to bring about healing. You need to try and stop seeing fever as something that *always* requires medicating. You need to try and stop judging how sick your child is in relation to how high their temperature is. You need to try and start supporting your child's miraculous immune system as it fights off illness and disease. That is quite a lot to ask, and I know that!

But it's not just me who is asking you to change how you perceive fever, it's the current scientific research too and most importantly it's our children who need us to stop. The British National Institute for Care Excellence (NICE) guidelines (2013) recommend not routinely treating children for a fever and only considering treating the fever if the "fever is associated with distress". They also recommend not treating fever to prevent febrile convulsions, as they have found "…no evidence that antipyretic drugs are effective in the prevention of febrile convulsions."

The American Academy of Pediatrics (AAP, 2011) has also issued guidelines on managing fevers in children that go even further, referring to the need to educate parents and families with regards to "fever phobia". They highlight the beneficial role fever plays in fighting infection and conclude that emphasis should be put on making the child comfortable and not on maintaining "normal" body temperature.

While some parents will argue that the reduction of fever does indeed enhance the comfort of the child, the AAP remains skeptical. They also highlight the risks posed from potential inaccurate dosing and that the side effects from these strong medications may outweigh the benefits. For example, paracetamol, in excess, has the potential to cause liver damage and death, and ibuprofen has the potential to cause gastric problems including ulcers and internal bleeding, as well as nose bleeds, blood clotting issues and potential problems with kidney function.

There is also plenty that can be done at home to make a child feel more comfortable without the need to interfere with a child's extraordinary and powerful immune system. Before we get onto the remedies, first let's examine why fever is so important and so beneficial for our children.

The Benefits of Fever

A fever is the body's way of fighting an infection either of bacterial or viral origin. Some of us may remember from school that increasing body temperature creates an inhospitable environment for both bacteria and viruses in which to replicate. You may also be aware that an increased temperature increases the body's metabolic rate, which means that the body does everything at high speed. So, the production of neutrophils, T-lymphocytes and interferon, (just a few of the extraordinary tools the body creates and uses to fight infection), happens faster and more prolifically at higher temperatures. There is a cascade reaction that floods the body with a multitude of healing and defensive cells, enzymes, hormones and chemicals. All this is triggered by the rise in body temperature.

Fevers are generally considered to not only protect the child, but also enhance and strengthen the immune system enabling optimal functioning. There is also growing evidence that the body recovers more quickly from viral infections with fewer complications if a fever is allowed to run its course. In particular, the use of Ibuprofen to relieve symptoms of chickenpox has been associated with prolonging the illness, worsening of symptoms such as itching, and development of a serious skin infection called necrotising fasciitis. Current medical advice is to avoid the use of Ibuprofen when treating chickenpox.

Immunologists are very familiar with how a fever reduces replication rates of viruses and bacteria, which has implications for the spread of disease throughout the general population. By treating a fever and lowering body temperature, the virus and bacteria are uninhibited and free to replicate as normal. This can increase the viral load in a child and means that when they sneeze, cough, vomit or pass stools, the amount of virus present in their bodily fluids (called viral shedding) is greater compared to that of a child who has a fever and therefore is inhibiting viral replication. This has implications for the spread of coughs, colds and particularly the flu. By reducing fever, we are potentially encouraging a greater proliferation of infectious illness.

Fever-reducing medication artificially increases the sense of wellbeing that a child feels and encourages social interaction in facilities such as schools and nurseries. This comes at a time when the child would ordinarily feel like withdrawing and resting. The increase in social interaction, combined with an increased viral load, enhances the ability of pathogens (disease-causing organisms), to be opportunistic and take advantage of a very favourable situation to infect a greater and greater population. Both points have been demonstrated experimentally and theoretically.

So just to recap: fever in a normally healthy child, caused by infection, enhances and strengthens the immune system's functioning. It can reduce the length of the illness compared to when fever-reducing medications are used; it can reduce the chances of further complications from illness when compared to using fever-reducing medication, and it can reduce the ability of viruses and bacteria to replicate, thus reducing viral load and limiting the spread of infectious disease.

An alternative view of the role of fever, and one frequently held by practitioners of complementary therapies, is that it is essentially the body cleansing itself and processing bodily challenges. Viruses and bacteria are seen as by-products of the cleansing process and not the cause of illness. The cause of disease is a combination of the individual's constitution and either poor diet, sleep, lifestyle, situational or emotional health. This is a truly *wholistic* view of an individual and how their body is choosing to express its dis-ease. When the load becomes too great on the individual, the body tries to re-calibrate, cleanse and balance itself to start afresh. This is when dis-ease becomes physically evident, and fever plays a vital role in the cleansing, replenishing and strengthening processes of the body.

There are a number of myths that feed the fear of fever, which many parents, grandparents, friends and the majority of medical professionals still believe to be true, despite evidence proving otherwise. The first myth to tackle is that there is a direct correlation between the increase in temperature of the child and the seriousness of the illness. This is absolutely not true and it is a dangerous assumption to make. Fever from an infection only ever indicates that the child's immune system is working. There are some non-threatening viruses such as Roseola and Hand, Foot and Mouth disease, which can cause very high spiking temperatures, and there are some extremely serious infections that barely cause a rise in temperature at all, such as Diphtheria. In some cases, a total lack of fever can indicate a very serious medical situation as the body is so overwhelmed by infection that it is unable to manifest a fever to fight it.

A fever caused by the body fighting an infection, is a simple, solitary indicator that a type of infection is present. There are other signs that are far more indicative of the level of seriousness of illness, such as respiratory distress (difficulty or effort involved in breathing), changes in consciousness and the general demeanour and behaviour of your child. The chapter on Assessing Your Child covers the symptoms that indicate a second opinion needs to be quickly sought from a medical professional.

The next myth is that if a fever is left untreated then it will continue to rise and very high fevers cause brain damage and inevitably seizures. There are several threads to this myth that need careful unpicking, and the best place to begin is to explain the difference between fevers caused by infection and fevers caused by external factors.

A fever caused by infection can rarely physically rise above 41.2 degrees

Celsius (or 106 degrees Fahrenheit), the body simply won't allow it. In fevers caused by external factors such as heatstroke (over-exertion in hot weather or due to over-dressing) or ingestion of substances such as poison or certain medications, then it is possible for these external factors, outside the body's control, to override the hypothalamus and cause the body temperature to rise above 41.2 degrees. The hypothalamus is the part of the brain that controls temperature regulation in the body through the release of hormones and chemical messengers. If this happens, then hyperthermia can cause neurological problems and impact on the brain. However, the body, without external factors overwhelming its internal thermostat, is naturally limited, and within this range a fever is usually not harmful.

Febrile seizures (convulsions linked to fever), do occur rarely, most often in children under the age of 5 years old, and children usually grow out of them. Febrile seizures are not considered to cause brain damage and are generally thought to be harmless to the child. Importantly they are also not considered to be determined by body temperature alone, rather the speed at which the temperature rises. Therefore, the administration of fever-reducing medicine is not advised by either the British NICE guidelines (2013) or the American Academy of Paediatrics (2011) for either the prevention or treatment of febrile seizures in children. Febrile seizures in childhood are also not considered to indicate a predisposition to developing epilepsy or seizures in adult life.

Having said that, witnessing a child having a seizure, especially for the first time, can be utterly terrifying and makes it very difficult to believe all that I have just written in the paragraph above. If your child has a seizure, or you witness a child having a seizure for the first time, make sure the child is safe by removing any objects they could harm themselves on, try not to restrict their movement, gently roll them onto their side if possible to avoid choking, stay with them and call the emergency services. If you can remember and are able, then it is always a good idea to try to time the length of a seizure, or ask a bystander to do this for you while you care for the child. It gives the paramedics and medical professionals some idea of the seriousness of a seizure and is useful information for them to help with treatment and diagnosis, as the chances are the child will have recovered by the time an ambulance arrives. Once the child has been diagnosed with febrile seizures, you can be reassured that no harm has occurred from the febrile seizure itself. The medical team will also advise and guide you on how best to manage fever in your child for the future.

Treating Fever

If you are new to managing a fever or illness without resorting to medication like paracetamol or ibuprofen, then you may feel anxious, worried and lacking in confidence. It is quite frightening to go against all that you have held to be true and to try something new. Your confidence will grow with practice, as your experience increases. Once you see that your child copes with fever, and you are able to ease their discomfort, so your trust and confidence in your own ability to nurse your child will develop. Your assessment skills will improve and you will recognise when you need to involve other health professionals, which should happen less and less often.

Then you will start to see the results as your child starts to show greater vitality and ability to fight off infection faster and with fewer complications. Perhaps the first fever you allow your child to experience un-medicated will last for five days, but the next may be three days. You will notice the child experiences shorter periods of fever and the body becomes increasingly efficient as the immune system is allowed to function unimpeded by conventional fever reducing drugs.

If you are extremely anxious, then it may be best to find a suitable healthcare practitioner who is familiar with managing fever without drugs. I would suggest finding one before your child gets unwell, and talk to them to ensure you are comfortable with their skills and knowledge. This way everything is in place for when the time comes.

There is also your doctor, nurse or A&E department if you are ever worried and feel your child needs urgent attention. Never hesitate to use these services as you will never regret having your little one looked at "just in case". You can also always revert to using fever-reducing medication as you did before if you lose your nerve or are very anxious. As I say, nothing in this book is dogma, and you know your child and your limitations best. Do what you feel you must, what you feel you are able and what you feel is best for your child and your family.

Please refer to the chapter on Assessing Your Child in conjunction with the relevant age-appropriate section in Part Two regarding fever management.

The Pattern of Fever

As the child's body reacts to an infection and the hypothalamus resets the body temperature to cause a fever, frequently a child will complain of feeling cold.

They may even shiver. Current medical advice does not advocate wrapping a child up to keep them warm if they are complaining of feeling cold, because that may raise a fever too quickly and cause a febrile seizure. My experience is that the body works very hard, even harder if it is struggling, to generate enough heat to reach the newly set temperature target. In my family, I help my children to gently warm up, but ONLY if they are showing signs like shivering and complaining of being cold.

I warm my children up by putting them to bed with a hot water bottle, (only if age appropriate), or giving them a warm bath and then putting them to bed. In my experience this treatment seems to help the body, and my children seem much more comfortable as a result.

Once the fever has reached its level and the child feels hot, then if it is necessary you can start treatments to make a child more comfortable. I would advise to only treat if or when the child shows signs of discomfort such as restlessness, lack of sleep, crying, grizzling or whimpering. If your child is coping with the fever, is resting and drinking well, then do not interfere with the extraordinary process your child's body is undertaking.

Your child will have a unique pattern of fever. I have two children and they both experience fever very differently. It is important that you observe the signs in your child so that you learn to recognise the beginning of a fever and get to know the treatments they respond to most. Below are my personal experiences with my two children, currently aged four and five years old.

Claudia: The first sign is that she will always complain of feeling cold even if the ambient temperature is warm and she is in appropriate clothing. She may go off her food slightly and she will start wandering around the house, or wherever we are, aimlessly, often being clumsy and bumping into things. She will ask for a warm bath, hot water bottle or go to bed and wrap herself up in as many layers of bedding as she can get her hands on. Her temperature rises very fast and always goes very high, as her 'normal' temperature is higher than the average 36.5 (97.7) degrees. Sometimes she feels sick or is sick because of the speed her temperature rises. Once her body reaches its target temperature to fight infection then she settles down. Because Claudia has a high "normal" temperature, a high fever for Claudia is usually around 40.3 – 41.0 degrees.

Her favourite treatments which she enjoys and help her to feel more comfortable are:

- Herbal tea in her special teapot and mug
- Appropriate remedies in her favourite pretty shot glasses
- A warm bath in the evening with cooling essential oils
- Being wrapped in a towel after the bath and having her feet and calves gently rubbed with lemon oil
- Having lemon socks applied
- Having a bath with rosemary oil the following morning after a feverish night
- Having fresh flowers in her room

Essentially Claudia likes to feel she is in a spa. She adores restful pampering and recovers at remarkable speed when she gets it. It is also a time when the two of us slow down and really strengthen our bond with each other. Spending time nurturing Claudia is very rewarding because she responds so well to it, and so quickly.

Joshua: He will be a bit grumpy and a bit tricky, nothing terribly obvious. He may complain of very vague symptoms or that he feels tired. He never has the initial feeling of being cold like Claudia. The first indication that he may have a fever is when I kiss his forehead and it feels unusually warm against my lips. I will normally take his temperature to confirm my suspicions. Joshua's temperature usually rises slower than Claudia's and his increase in temperature has only made him sick once. Although everyone's breathing rate increases with a fever, (all metabolic processes increase), Joshua's seems to be even more marked, certainly more than Claudia. He is more restless when he sleeps with a fever and can wake frequently so sleeps with me when he is unwell.

His favourite treatments that help him to sleep peacefully and rest and recuperate quickly are:

- Herbal tea in his own mug and teapot. Joshua can drink a lot of herbal tea. He really feels it's medicine so it doesn't seem to matter what it tastes like, as long as it's sweetened with honey or maple syrup
- Joshua likes a bath in the evening with thyme and cooling herbs or oils
- He loves a slow morning bath with rosemary oil

- Usually, he wants to eat only raw fruit
- He likes to have a bed made up on the sofa so he can watch *Thomas the Tank Engine* and doze off having a cuddle
- Lemon socks definitely help him sleep well and in a calmer fashion
- He loves being read to.

Joshua is much less treatment-focused and really needs TLC and company more than anything. He is a real trooper and needs close observation to make sure he isn't pushing himself to do too much too soon. I have learnt from experience that he takes longer to recuperate and convalesce if he doesn't rest properly during the initial phase of illness.

So, I have two children, each with a very different pattern of fever, and different ideas about what helps them to feel better. I should imagine your child or children will be completely different to my children. This is the remarkable thing about the human race; we are all unique in how we experience both health and illness. Observational skills are key for any medical practitioner and especially any parent. This is doubly true if you have a baby who is not communicating verbally yet. Observation and patience are vital, and the more those skills are practised, the quicker you will find the remedies that suit and work for your child.

At the end of the book is a section for *Notes* (not on the Kindle edition) for you to write and make your observations about your child's health, the remedies you've tried and any positive and negative reactions to them. As your child grows it will become increasingly clear to you what works and suits their own individual constitution. Also don't be afraid to talk to others, read books and ask advice because, as Juliette de Bairacli Levy once wrote:

"The Wise Woman seeks help from many sources, including her inner guidance, trusted friends and trained healers, in addition to the words written here."

As a final note, many different cultures and branches of medicine consider fever in a child to be a pre-cursor to a developmental leap. Frequently parents report that their child, once recovered from the fever, starts crawling or walking or talking, or reaches some other developmental milestone. That is not to say that if a fever is treated with paracetamol or ibuprofen the child doesn't develop, but they do seem to lack both the dramatic leap, and the emergence from illness with renewed vigour and vitality. Much of this is anecdotal, of course, but hopefully of interest to some of you. Theories and observations from medical practitioners and systems far older and wiser than the current conventional model often have a different take on the role of illness, and can sometimes have deep wisdom to share with us if we are only willing to listen.

Chapter Two

The Healing Environment

Ideally the healing environment will be within the child's home, where he or she feels comfortable and secure, and most importantly, cared for. However, any place can be turned into a healing environment provided there is an adult present who can tend to the child with a nurturing and caring manner. If an ill child feels safe and supported, their adrenaline and cortisol levels, (stress hormones which suppress the immune system), will reduce, enabling the body to rest properly and the immune system to function optimally.

Light

At night time, it is a good idea to keep light very low-level, but enough to give comfort to the child when they wake and for you to see properly when checking and tending to them. A night-light is a good idea, but also the soft pink glow of a natural Himalayan salt lamp works well and has the added benefit of helping to reduce allergens and irritants in the air. A Himalayan salt lamp can create a lovely fresh environment, perfect for aiding rest and recuperation, while also providing much needed light at an adequately low level to not disturb sleep, but high enough to give sufficient night time visibility.

Air

Aim to freshen the air in a sick room at least once a day, preferably in the morning. The ideal would be in the morning and again in the evening before settling for the night. It keeps the air circulating, the germs at bay and the oxygen replenished. Psychologically, a child (or adult for that matter), always 'feels' better when put to bed in clean bedclothes, in a well-aired room. It can help a child settle faster in the evening and seems to improve their general energy levels and vitality.

When the weather is cold or a child's temperature is rising and they feel cold and shivery then have a window open just a fraction, a gap as small as half a centimetre is enough to slowly change the air of the room over the day. If it is too cold for a window to be open while the child is in the room, move the child to another bedroom or the sofa, or bathe them for a while as you change or freshen bedding and give their sick room a good airing by opening the windows.

If the weather is hot, and you have a child with a fever, it is tempting to allow a breeze from a window or electric fan to blow directly onto them. Please try to avoid this as it may cool the body too quickly. Rapid cooling can cause a 'shock' response, inducing nausea and vomiting or violent shivering, as the body redoubles its efforts to raise and maintain a fever. Instead, open the window wide but keep blinds and curtains closed to help keep the room cool and prevent draughts blowing directly onto the child. An electric fan can be used but have it directed away from the child as this will allow the child to be cooled by circulating air rather than being blasted directly by the fan. If the room is really hot then fill a bowl with water and place it in the freezer. Once the water is frozen, place the bowl in front of the fan so the air is cooled by the ice and is circulated around the room. If you do use this method then take care when having water near an electrical appliance and ensure that the fan is not likely to tip into the water. It's the best alternative if air conditioning isn't available and this method can cool a room by a couple of degrees if done consistently.

Using essential oils to help cleanse the air within the home and encourage rest and healing is also a good idea. Suggestions for essential oil blends to cleanse the air that are antibacterial or antiviral can be found below:

Antibacterial oil blend
one *drop Basil oil*
two *drops Lemon oil*
one *drop Eucalyptus oil*

Antiviral oil blend
one *drop Eucalyptus or Tea Tree oil*
one *drop Thyme oil*
two *drops Lime oil*

Mix your chosen blend together and apply to an aromatherapy vaporiser or diffuser according to the manufacturer's instructions. If possible, try to use either an Aroma-Stream Vaporiser or an essential oil diffuser. Alternatively, you can blend the oils in a small bottle with a spray top, then add 20 ml of water to the oil blend, shake well and spray into the air around the room like an air freshener. All of these avoid the use of candles, which can be a hazard if left unattended. Of course, all essential oils and vaporisers should be kept well out of the reach of children.

Airing and cleaning the wards and rooms of sick patients were the first basic and simple steps the nurses in the Crimean War took to prevent the spread of disease, reduce infection and increase patient survival rates. If done properly, it is a very simple way to impact on the atmosphere of a room and increase patient comfort. Just make sure that the child is kept out of direct draughts, is covered with bedding appropriate to the time of year and temperature of the room, and that they don't get cold.

Food and Fluids

Food is often described in terms of comfort, nourishment and soul-replenishing qualities. Food clearly has emotional implications and is used for spiritual purposes too, such as marking religious festivals, offering food to gods and goddesses, or the literal breaking of bread during worship. So, when preparing food for a child who has a tentative appetite and is beginning to recover from an illness, it is a demonstration of love, care and a desire to nurture and nourish, to replenish the child physically and emotionally.

I have tried to reflect this need in my chapter Recipes for Recovery; however, the recipes may not fit in with your personal lifestyle, religious views or the child's unique preferences. If that is the case then just be mindful that any food you prepare for a child who is convalescing should be of small portions, nourishing and tempting on an emotional and physical level. If we reflect on our own childhood there will be specific foods we remember being fed when ill or recovering, and just thinking of these foods often reawakens feelings of nurture and comfort.

In contrast, a sickening or acutely unwell child will almost always be off their food. This is quite normal, and indeed advocated by some branches of complementary medicine, where fasting whilst unwell is believed to be essential to the healing process. Food in this stage should be kept very simple and often in a form that is easy to digest such as juices, soups, jellies and purees. Herbal teas and infusions are also packed full of vitamins and minerals and are nourishing for both body and mind. I have included some ideas and suggestions in the chapter Recipes During Illness.

Fluids however are different; they are essential in helping the child through the process of healing, and a dehydrated child is a very unwell child indeed.

Having said that, force-feeding fluids using syringes, bottles, cups and so on, is counterproductive and carries the very real risk of the child aspirating (inhaling) fluid into the lungs. Dehydration is covered in more detail in a separate chapter called Assessing Your Child, but when encouraging your child to take fluid, frequent small sips is the key to helping your child remain comfortable. Buying some small, attractive 'shot' glasses, typically used for schnapps or liqueur, or espresso cups, and filling them only halfway with filtered water or a small amount of herbal tea or diluted juice, can help encourage a child to drink. Firstly, the amount looks tiny so is not daunting for the child, and the design of the glasses often encourages the child to 'down it' in one gulp. The glasses are small enough and sturdy enough for little hands to cope with as well as having novelty value. Giving a child a small amount of fluid using this method every 15-20 minutes can really help to keep hydration levels adequate. Sometimes presenting the fluid in a different or unique way is enough to encourage a few sips.

If your child has been weaned, then including fluid in food is a good way of increasing uptake. Please see the Recipe Chapters for specific ideas, but all fruits contain water as do vegetables. Offering a child prepared raw fruit, especially berries, as well as fruit purees and soups will all help to boost fluid intake.

The main thing is not to panic. Don't force-feed your child fluids, offer and encourage regular small sips. Monitor your child using the guidelines in the Dehydration Chapter if you have concerns, and always consult a medical professional if you are worried that your child may be dehydrated.

Clothing and Bedding

Clothing and bedding should all be made of natural fibres, preferably cotton, to allow the skin to breathe and for easy washing. Pyjamas and night clothes should reflect the time of year and the temperature and comfort of the child.

It is always advisable to keep the child covered with a sheet as a minimum because it enables a more measured way for the body to adjust to changes in temperature.

As for babies who are too young for bedding, then a thin, pure cotton summer sleeping bag is ideal for a baby with a fever who is hot. Inside the sleeping bag the parent can dress the baby appropriately. Babies struggle to regulate their own body temperature so extra vigilance is required to ensure the baby doesn't get overheated or chilled.

If a baby requires a thicker, warmer sleeping bag, then I recommend Bambino Merino sleeping bags. They are made with cotton and merino: a fine, soft wool, which is very thin and is a natural thermo-regulator. It is machine washable and regulates the body temperature of babies superbly; a truly miraculous and natural material, used by arctic explorers and parents alike.

Screen Time

Ipads, computers, phones and tablets, in fact anything with a digital screen, is not recommended for a child who is ill with a fever. The images are too stimulating and the digital light emitted from these screens inhibits the brain from switching off and resting properly. An alternative is old television shows that are gentle and slow, and have not been filmed digitally, that children can watch if they really need a distraction. In our house we save them for when the kids are ill, so the DVDs still retain their novelty value. Firm favourites are *Ivor the Engine*, *Button Moon*, *Thomas the Tank Engine* (the older ones read by Ringo Starr), *Bagpuss*, *The Moomins*, *Kipper Classic Collection*, *Here Comes A... Fire Engine!*

The best thing for a child who is ill is rest. Resting in their bed is the ideal, in a quiet and calm environment. Picking some fresh flowers or attractive foliage from the garden and placing it in a small vase within the eye line of the child, (but not within physical reach) gives them something to gaze at while resting. Most children will sleep when they are unwell and are allowed to have a fever.

Books are also great. The child can either look at them alone or be read to. Reading to a sick child is a lovely quiet way to comfort the child and allow them to feel nurtured. It is also a good way to spend time with the child so you can assess their responses, pallor, comfort and general condition. Assessing a child during such a calm and quiet activity means that it can be done without the child really noticing they are being observed, and this way you can gain a more accurate picture of their state of health.

Talking books or radio programs like Cbeebies Radio are also beneficial; they provide quiet and calm entertainment without engaging too many senses for the child. Having said all of that, you know your child best, and if keeping your child calm and rested requires all manner of screen interaction and noise, then that's fine too. The end frequently justifies the means when it comes to children, and it is, after all, a matter of personal choice and parental preference.

Preparation

As a mother, I have learnt the hard way that preparation is key to managing an unwell child in a calm and confident manner. I don't know why a child always seems to get really ill on a Friday or Saturday night, when the shops are all shut, the GP has gone home and you have run out of all medicines and remedies that could possibly help. You may find the cupboard is bare except for a horribly out-of-date sachet of nasty blackcurrant-flavour rehydration powder... We have all been there I think.

At the risk of sounding like a total control freak, I plan ahead for the Autumn and Winter, I buy or make the remedies and medicines I know I will most likely need and a few extra just to make sure I've got most bases covered, and then I wait...

Also put some preparation in for yourself. Make sure you have a couple of ready-meals in the freezer, ideally ones that are just as good to eat cold as hot, and take very little time to cook. In our house pizza with a ready-made salad, any sort of pasta and ready-made sauce, soup with bread, beans on toast and scrambled egg seem to work well. Once a poorly child has settled you never know how long you have until the next bout of coughing/vomiting/crying/comforting will occur, so nutrition (and it's a case of needs must rather than ideal or optimal!) needs to be able to be prepared quickly and eaten fast, likely in shifts, and still palatable once it's cold.

Small glass shot glasses, or baby-weaning cups (www.babycup.co.uk), are a brilliant way to administer medicines during the night. If your child needs cough syrup or homeopathic remedies, then they can be measured out and diluted in a small amount of water in a shot glass or small cup before bed and left where they can easily be reached by an adult in the night to give to the child as and when needed. This sort of preparation means no fumbling around in the dark trying to pour medicine onto a teaspoon and getting covered in a sticky mess, no tipping a pill into the lid of a jar hoping you have got just the one, or trying to count 10, no more squinting in the darkness to try and see the measurements on an oral syringe you are drawing up. This way the work is already done, everything is lined up and to hand when needed.

If you have a small baby and use oral syringes for giving medicine, then these can all be drawn up in advance before bedtime, (you can ask your pharmacist for extra oral syringes or order online). Alternatively, you can dissolve all homeopathic remedies or herbal remedies into a small amount of water in shot glasses ready to draw up into the syringe when required.

If the difference between remedies and medicines isn't obvious due to colour or amount, then always make sure you clearly label the medicines you have pre-prepared. Write the name on a piece of paper and put the glass or syringe on top of it, or stick a post-it note on it. Just make sure you come up with a way to ensure you know what you are administering. And always make sure all medicines are out of reach of children.

Chapter Three

How To Use The Remedies In This Book

Homeopathy

Homeopathy is a very gentle form of medicine, ideal for use in children due to a lack of dangerous side effects. Homeopathy is safe to use in newborns and the elderly and everyone in between. There are different strengths of remedy available and different schools of thought about how remedies should be taken. The suggestions in this book are by no means hard and fast rules; please feel free to explore and research this form of medicine for yourself. Homeopathy has detractors, mainly from science fundamentalists, but I would suggest keeping an open mind. It will not do any harm, and a worst-case scenario is that it will do nothing. The best-case scenario is that you may have discovered a gentle form of medicine that is a viable and effective way to treat your whole family.

I am not a purist when it comes to homeopathy and treating an acutely sick child at 3am! I will frequently be found dissolving three different homeopathic remedies, or maybe more, into some water in a small shot glass ready for my child to take. I do combine remedies, and I suggest you do too if you are trying to find something to help your child and you can't quite decide which individual remedy to use.

Homeopathy prescribes a specific remedy depending on the characteristics or symptoms the patient displays. So, for instance, your child may have a fever, be red in the face and very restless and extremely thirsty. These particular symptoms will point to a specific remedy. Having a fever, being listless, calm and looking washed out, indicate the need for a different remedy, despite fever being a common factor. It can be quite difficult trying to find the best fit between symptom picture and remedy when it's the middle of the night and your child needs something NOW, and you have limited experience, knowledge, or sleep deprivation has turned your brain to mush.

There are also recipes for combination remedies for some illnesses, and these can be made up by a homeopathic pharmacy for you. There are three addresses of reputable and well known pharmacies in the UK in the Resources section; however, you may know of another one or have one near to you, in which case please support them.

Homeopathic remedies tend to work quite fast if you have chosen the correct remedy. Give the remedy frequently to start, up to every 15-30 minutes for the first 4 doses, and then as and when needed (usually once or twice a day). If no change is observed over 24 hours, or sooner if you feel necessary, then change the remedy and try something else. My advice would be to stop giving a remedy when improvement occurs, or symptoms change. Take your time to allow the healing process to occur, and just quietly assess and observe the child you are treating.

If you are ever unsure or feel you need more expertise in making a choice of remedy for your child, I would recommend seeing a qualified homeopath. You can find them recommended by word of mouth, in the yellow pages, on the internet, or through a governing body such as the Society of Homeopaths (SoH) in the UK. In the United Kingdom, there is also the Homeopathy Helpline, which, although it has a premium rate call charge, very quickly (usually in less than 10 minutes), gives very accurate and useful advice. They are open from 9am until midnight seven days a week, which is perfect for the out-of-hours panic that most parents have experienced at least once in their lives.

Two companies called *Helios* and *Ainsworth* make their own homeopathic kits that include the most common and useful remedies likely to be used at home. They also do a First Aid Kit, Childbirth Kit and a Travel Kit. This is a handy and cost effective way to have a good and varied selection of remedies to hand at home for emergencies and illness. Included in each kit is advice for appropriate remedy selection and administration, so even a total beginner can use the kits with confidence. Both Ainsworth and Helios are excellent at sending remedies out extremely promptly when ordered over the phone, and during office hours they also have homeopaths and pharmacists on hand to advise.

N.B. Never touch homeopathic medicines with your hands or fingers. Remedies are sprayed onto the lactose-based pillules, tablets or granules, so physically touching them removes the remedy from the pillule. Always tip the pills out into the lid of the remedy container or onto a clean teaspoon to count them out, before tipping them directly into water, juice or the mouth of the child.

Administering Homeopathic Medicines

Babies – I would usually advise buying homeopathic remedies in pillule form (a tiny pill, shaped like a small ball). To administer the remedy to a baby, you can dissolve a pillule in a small amount of cooled, boiled water. Once dissolved draw up one to two ml into an oral syringe or dropper and administer slowly, always into the inside cheek of a baby, never directly to the back of the throat. This slows the fluid down, allowing it to trickle to the back of the throat, triggering the swallowing reflex in a small baby. If fluid is administered directly to the back of the throat the swallowing reflex may not work in time and there is a risk that the fluid may go into the lungs.

A small feed bottle of cooled boiled water can also be made up with remedies dissolved in the water and the baby given frequent sips. This is especially easy and convenient during nighttime administration if your baby is already feeding from a bottle.

Another way is to tip a pillule onto a clean teaspoon, place another clean teaspoon over the top and crush the pillule into a powder between the two spoons. Then gently scrape the powder into the baby's mouth, or even onto the mother's nipple before nursing. The powder can also be tipped onto a sterilized bottle teat, or if your baby uses a pacifier, you can dip the dummy into the sweet remedy powder.

Some remedies are in an alcohol base, either ethanol or brandy, such as Bach Flower remedies. You can put the advised number of drops directly into formula that has been made up for the baby, or place drops into a small amount of water and allow to sit for approximately 15 minutes, as the majority of the alcohol will evaporate. Then the remedy/water mix can be drawn up into a syringe and administered into the inside of the baby's cheek very slowly.

Ages 18 months and up – Use any of the previously mentioned techniques if they work for you, or put remedies directly in the child's Sippy Cup, fill with water or diluted juice and allow the child to sip as required.

At this age a child would usually allow a pillule to be tipped directly into their mouth from the lid or cap of the remedy bottle. This is a really fast and simple way of administering remedies. Never tip any alcohol-based remedies directly into a child's mouth though; always dilute in water first.

The strengths I recommend are either 6C or 30C, which appear on the label of the remedies, or you can ask your homeopath, homeopathic pharmacist or Health Food shop assistant for further explanation and specific advice and suggestions.

Herbs

Herbs come in a vast variety of forms; syrups, tinctures, teas, infusions, glycerites, oils, vinegars – you name it, you can get a herb in it! I will mainly recommend teas, infusions, tinctures and glycerites, and I will explain dosage and give instructions according to the age of the child. The suggestions in this book are mild and gentle; a qualified medical herbalist who can actually see your child and examine them will be able to contribute more specific and bespoke medicines and recommendations.

Herbal tinctures are a concentrated way of administering herbal medicine. They have an advantage over herbal teas because they are easily disguised and diluted in water or juices because so much less of the medicine is required for a therapeutic effect. They usually contain alcohol, but some herbalists and herbal pharmacies do special tinctures for children in a base of vegetable glycerin which avoid the use of alcohol (these are known as glycerites). The quantities of alcohol are so minute when diluted that many parents are not bothered by its presence. My personal preference is for teas, but if you have a child who struggles to take herbal tea, then a tincture or glycerite may be the way forward. Tinctures and glycerites also have a long shelf life, which is an advantage for the medicine cabinet.

Please see the Resources section of the book for suggested outlets that make excellent quality tinctures and glycerites. If you have recommendations, or are lucky enough to have a local herbalist or herbal pharmacy, then please support them. Alternatively, you can make your own, and there are plenty of wonderful wise women who have published books with recipes and step-by-step instructions on how to do this. Again, I refer you to the Resources section where I have listed my favourite authors, although there are many others.

When herbal teas are suggested in this book, for ease of use I would suggest using tea bags. All the teas can be found in bags, and can be bought from most Health food shops, and certainly ordered online. One of my favourite brands is Hambleden Herbs, who make organic teas with unbleached bags and labels. I have always found them to be of the highest quality, and a good medicinal strength. Floradix also make wonderful quality organic herbal tea, and I use their Thyme and Sage daily. My other favourite brand of tea is one I managed to get in Australia and was called Organic India. Their Chai blends with Tulsi were utterly delicious. Other brands I use are Yogi Tea, Healtheries, Dr Stuart's, and the hardest one to get hold of, but arguably one of the best, Sidroga.

If you prefer, and have the time, then growing and harvesting your own herbs is very satisfying, as is foraging in the countryside for them. There are many books on how best to do this and how to store your herbs for the winter; my favourite books are listed in the Resources section.

Most of the herbs I suggest grow very happily in the kitchen garden, and you may have several of them in yours already. Feel free to snip them off and use them. The most common and useful herbs that are frequently mentioned in this book are rosemary, thyme, lavender and lemon balm. If you feel daunted at the prospect of using common herbs as medicine as opposed to culinary seasoning, please be reassured; women have been in charge of the household medicinal kitchen for centuries. The more you use these herbs the more confident you will grow, and you will be amazed at the healing power of these common, kitchen garden plants.

Alternatively, you can buy your herbs already dried and loose, or as tinctures and glycerites from many Natural Health shops and they can give good advice too. There are also a few traditional herbal apothecaries dotted around the UK, and in other countries too (I found a fantastic one tucked away in Raglan, New Zealand). Here you will find highly skilled and qualified herbalists who can create bespoke blends of herbs for many conditions. In the UK, the best I have found so far is Botanica Medica in Esher. They give free advice and are a wonderful resource if you want to find out more about herbs. They offer guided herbal walks and also send herbal blends and books by post throughout the country, so don't worry if you don't live near Esher! There are many, many wonderful herbalists and herb retailers, my list is not exhaustive and my opinion is just one of many! Please explore and find your own treasure troves and share them.

Brewing and Administering Herbal Teas and Baths

Herbal Baths

Unless stated otherwise, the following instructions would be my preference for creating a medicinal herbal bath. Individual measurements and blends of herbs can be found in the appropriate section.

You can of course allow teas to brew for longer than I have suggested. Also, as your child grows up please feel free to use any suggested herbal baths that are in the sections for younger children. As your confidence and knowledge grows, your own research may lead you to other combinations of herbs outside this book. Every child is unique and will respond in their own way to different treatments and plants so I would encourage exploring and experimentation within the parameters of your own knowledge and expertise.

Pour a litre of boiling water into a bowl or jug, and add the suggested measurements of herbs (either fresh, dried or teabags) to the freshly boiled water. Cover the vessel and allow the herbs to brew for 30 minutes, or up to an hour. Run a bath for the baby and add the brewed tea to the bath water. Squeeze every last drop out of the herbs, and if you have used loose herbs then strain the tea through a sieve lined with a muslin, as you pour the tea into the bath. Don't worry about any tiny bits of herb floating in the bath unless it is likely to end up in your child's mouth or eye, or blocking the plug and drain.

Check the temperature of the bath once the herbal tea has been added. The bath should be the normal temperature you use for your baby or child; if you dip your elbow in the water it should feel warm. Don't allow the bath to be any cooler or hotter than normal.

Allow the baby to sit in the tea bath for 10-15 minutes, or until your child has had enough. While your baby is in the bath, gently bathe their body with the herbal tea bath using a flannel or your cupped hands. Don't wet the baby's hair if the baby has a temperature or is unwell.

Ensure windows and doors are closed whilst bathing so that any medicinal oils evaporating in the steam of the bath water can be inhaled by your little one.

If your child is not well enough for a bath, or simply doesn't want a bath, the herbal brew can be added to a basin or bowl, and the child can be washed with a flannel. If the child is well enough to get out of bed and be washed in the bathroom, then that is fine. Ensure you have fresh clothes to hand so they don't get chilled whilst being washed. If necessary your child can be washed in bed, like an old-fashioned bed bath, and for those unfamiliar with the process I explain it in the chapter of the book on Practical Nursing Therapies At Home.

Making a Herbal Tea

To anyone living in England, making a cup of tea probably comes as naturally as breathing I should think, so explaining how to brew herbal tea does seem a bit ridiculous. However, as I stated at the beginning of this book, I am assuming there may be someone reading this who has never brewed tea in their life before. Equally there may be nervous parents who need a bit of reassurance. Forgive me if this section of the book is too simplistic for you, and feel free to skip it if you feel confident in this area.

Dosages for tea can be found in the relevant section as can suggestions for blends and combinations.

There is a general rule of thumb regarding brewing times for herbal tea that is going to be drunk (as opposed to bathed in), that I can share with you. Flowers generally should be brewed for no longer than 15 to 20 minutes; any longer can make the brew taste bitter. Leaves can be brewed for longer – up to eight to twelve hours, although this will taste truly medicinal and strong! And roots can be brewed for up to 24 hours to fully extract medicinal qualities. I don't recommend such lengthy brewing in this book, as the tea needs to be pleasant to taste for children, and you can certainly get medicinal benefits from a weaker tea.

Also, consuming herbal tea is a way of helping an unwell child maintain adequate hydration levels and feel comforted and nurtured. Better to sip a mild tea frequently than a strong medicinal one rarely – and find it revolting to boot!

Many of the teas suggested in this book can be given as a single tea or combined together. Experiment to see which tea your child finds most palatable, and if the tea needs to be sweetened then use a small amount of fruit juice or maple syrup if your baby is under one years old, as honey is not recommended. However, honey is perfectly acceptable as a sweetener after one year of age.

Freshly brewed, cooled tea can also be used as part of the fluid component used to make up formula if your baby is formula fed. If your baby is exclusively breast fed, then the mother can drink the teas freely throughout the day (unless stated otherwise) and the beneficial medicinal effects can be absorbed into the breast milk and passed to your baby through breastfeeding. As a mother, it is perfectly safe for you to sweeten your own herbal teas with honey as it poses no risk to your baby via breastmilk.

Consuming herbal tea as a breastfeeding mother for the benefit of your baby is a wonderful and comforting way to administer herbal medicine, and in many instances, it has the added advantage of benefitting the mother too!

- For babies less than six months old I would suggest brewing tea in a sterilised bottle or glass. For children older than six months, a clean teapot or mug is fine.
- Brew herbal tea using a teaspoon of either fresh or dried herbs, or a teabag and approximately 250 ml (or one normal sized mug) of freshly boiled water. If using loose herbs, ensure they are either contained in a mesh metal 'tea infuser' or that you have a tea strainer to filter out the herbs before administering the tea to a child.
- Allow the herbs to steep in the boiled water, preferably covered, for the specified amount of time and then allow to cool.
- Once cool, the correct dosage of tea can either be added to formula as part of the liquid component, or the cooled tea can be mixed in with fruit juice, sweetened with a dash of maple syrup or honey if appropriate, or given as a simple tea either direct from the bottle, or using an oral syringe or a medicinal dropper in the correct dosage.
- When using an oral syringe please be very careful as tea is a thin liquid, and will come out of the syringe quickly. Administer the tea very slowly through the syringe into the side of the baby's cheek.

Alternatively, you can encourage your baby to take the tea directly off a teaspoon or from a small medicine cup. You may have to use a mixture of these methods of administration or invent some of your own! If you have any great success stories, please let me know so we can spread the word and help other parents.

The tea can be kept refrigerated in the sterile bottle or glass for a maximum of four hours before a fresh brew is required. For older children (from six months old), tea can be kept in a clean teapot or other covered jug or vessel, either in the fridge or on the side for up to six hours.

I have a small jug or teapot for my children that contains slightly more than an average mugful of tea. I brew their tea in there in the morning, and I find the teapot is easy for me to go to throughout the day once the tea has cooled and it is also an easy way for me to keep track of how much they are drinking.

Sweetened tea can also be made into ice-lollies for older toddlers, and babies can have frozen tea as ice cubes put into a teething/weaning bag – a small mesh bag attached to a dummy-like contraption, that helps eliminate the risk of choking on foods. There are several types, but the one I have experience of is called the *Munchkin Fresh Food Feeder*. It can get messy, but the inventor was a genius! This cools the child as well as encouraging the child to take the herbal brew.

As a parent, you will need to exercise your own judgment and not leave the child unsupervised whilst sucking on an ice cube or ice-lolly. Alternatively, there are also recipes for Herbal Tea Jelly and Herbal Iced Tea in the Recipes During Illness chapter.

Essential Oils

Essential oils are obtained from plants, flowers, seeds, barks or resins, usually by the process of distillation. Any essential oil will consist of highly concentrated aromatic and medicinal compounds, and by using only a very small amount of essential oil, it is possible to experience the benefits of these compounds. Less is always more when using this form of medicine and never use more than the recommended dose without seeking advice from a qualified Aromatherapist first. As with any medicine, always keep the oils out of reach of children.

Essential oils are very potent and should never be used undiluted on children's skin. In this book, they will mainly be used in baths, as inhalations, or topically, but only when heavily diluted. I will provide instructions according to the age of the child and the specific oil used in the relevant section of this book.

Essential oils can seem expensive, but it is worth buying the best quality you can afford, because a little goes a long way, and the better the quality, the more effective the oil. I like to buy mine from Neal's Yard in the UK, because they offer organic versions of oils, and their quality can be guaranteed. They also have a large enough network to ensure a good turnover in essential oils, which means those I buy should be nice and fresh (hopefully!). There are many suppliers though, so it is definitely worth shopping around.

In Conclusion

I have tried to avoid recommending anything too obscure or difficult to get hold of. I feel extremely lucky to live in the UK, where most things are available with just a little time spent searching on the internet or from local shops.

I am almost obsessive about independent Natural Health Food Shops and visit any that I happen to drive or walk past. My husband and children have been dragged into them all over the world, and sometimes, if I'm really impressed and want to remember them I take photos and make notes. I have a sort of scrap book on Health Food shops, pharmacies and apothecaries from all over the world that I have loved. The people who work in them and run them are often the most interesting aspect of the shop. I always ask lots of questions, because you can always learn something new, and I enjoy hearing differing views and opinions from my own. It keeps me on my toes! Make use of any you have nearby, they are a valuable asset and resource to any community and are full of people wanting to share their knowledge with you. Almost everything I mention in this book should be available in one near to you.

I have also tried to include recipes where you can have a go making a few of the remedies yourself, and I really hope you try. There's nothing nicer in midwinter than cracking open some Elderberry or Rosehip syrup that you made in the summer or autumn. My children adore 'making potions' and medicines for our medicine chest. Going for walks, picking ingredients and creating something nourishing and health-giving is something they have helped me with as soon as they could walk. It's a surefire way to get a child to take medicine if they have been thoroughly involved in the production process.

Chapter Four

Assessing Your Child

I always find it useful to be able to look at facts and figures in black and white so I can see for myself that my child is not getting any worse, or is starting to turn the corner and get better. Sometimes it is the small signs that would ordinarily be missed that can indicate the very beginnings of improvement or deterioration. In this section I will start by talking you through the physiological signs medical professionals observe, why we look for them and what they can potentially indicate, and how to observe these signs so we know that we are getting an accurate reflection of health.

At the end of this chapter you will find some tables and charts, (I refer to them as 'tools'), to help you assess your child and record your findings if you need to.

You do not need to use the assessment tools to diagnose your child or speculate about prognosis. Please do not use them as a substitute for the opinion of a trained health professional. The tools are merely a guide to give you peace of mind when you need it or alert you to the fact that your child may need medical care or intervention. These assessment tools are designed to be straightforward to use and give valuable information to parents and health professionals. However, first let's start by thinking about what physiological signs we will be observing, why we observe them and how to do it accurately so they are meaningful.

Observing the Breathing Rate
(Respiratory Rate, abbreviated to RR)

I find this the most indicative physiological observation to monitor. It is often the first physiological symptom that will change to indicate improvement or deterioration in both children and adults. It is easy to assess and when I first see a patient I will always immediately notice how they are breathing. The speed, effort and how a person breathes can say a lot about how they are in terms of their health and wellbeing. Changes in both the rate and how a child is breathing are certainly not to be ignored, and for parents who worry about a child developing meningitis or sepsis, it is the child's breathing that will change well before any other symptoms, such as a rash, appear.

How to Assess the Breathing Rate
(Respiratory Rate / RR)

If a child is old enough to be aware of what you are doing, then it can prove difficult to get a true impression of a child's breathing rate. The child must not be aware that their breathing is being assessed. I usually pretend that I am taking their pulse, but although I am holding their wrist I am in fact counting their breaths and watching their chest rise and fall. Another way is to watch television or look at a book with your child, have your arm around them so that your hand is on their tummy or chest so you can feel the rise and fall of each breath. By far the most accurate way to count a breathing rate is while they are asleep!

Either the timer on a mobile phone needs to be set for a minute, or the pinger on the oven or watch. If you set a timer, then you can just concentrate on counting breaths until you hear a minute has passed. One breath is counted as an inspiration and expiration, so breathing in and out is one count.

Once you have counted the number of breaths your child has taken in a minute, it is time to look at *how* they are breathing. Are they breathing through their mouth or their nose? Are they making any noise, like grunting noises? Are they using accessory muscles when they breathe, such as sucking in the muscles/skin between their ribs when they breathe in, or the skin around the collarbones or base of the throat? Are their nostrils flaring when they breathe in, known as nasal flaring? Can you hear noises as they inhale or exhale? What colour is your child's skin? Is their skin pale and clammy or pink and warm? Does their breathing look easy and relaxed to you? Is your child quiet and still because of the effort they are putting into breathing, or are they still pottering around, interacting and responding?

A fever will always increase the rate of breathing, as it increases the speed of most bodily processes. This is normal and will usually manifest as a breathing rate in the upper ranges of normal, or perhaps just outside normal ranges by a breath or two. Concerns should be raised if the child increases their *effort* visibly to accommodate faster breathing. When assessing your child, it is important to take into account how far out of the 'normal' ranges they are, and for how long they have been outside the normal ranges. Looking at *how* a child is breathing will give a picture of general health and energy levels. If their breathing worsens, especially with regards to effort, then it is an excellent indicator that their general health may be worsening too, as they could be getting tired and it is time to get them assessed by a medical professional.

Observing the Circulation

Circulation (the movement of blood and fluids around the body) is important to assess in a child with a fever because it helps contribute to the general picture of whether a child's health is recovering, is static, or is deteriorating. Circulation is what gives white people their pinkish colour in health, and keeps our hands, feet and body warm to touch. In ill health, circulation plays an important role in carrying specific blood cells, chemicals and hormones to the site of infection within the body. It responds to and carries the cascade of hormonal information around the body so that an immune response can be launched. The body can prioritise aspects of circulation and can direct blood flow to just the major organs, leaving hands, feet and all extremities cold and slow to fill up with blood.

The colour of a child's skin is dependent on circulation. When a child has a fever and their face is bright red and hot, their blood is at the surface of their skin turning it bright pink/red in an effort to cool the body down. If a child appears very pale, perhaps with a bluish tinge to their skin, this can mean that either there is a lack of oxygen turning the red blood cells 'red' or there is a lack of circulation to the skin. The skin can also appear mottled, which is another sign that circulation to the skin surface is being withdrawn and being utilised deeper into the organs of the body. Similarly, the non-blanching rash of meningitis and/or sepsis appearing on the skin is actually where the capillaries in the skin are leaking giving a similar appearance to small blood blisters under the skin. This happens when the body has literally gone into 'overdrive' fighting infection and is in a life-threatening situation.

The temperature of a child's skin is also important to note, particularly when examining hands, feet, arms and legs. It is usually by touch that a parent or carer is first alerted that a child may have a fever, and the gentle touch of a parent, through a cuddle, hand hold or foot rub can quietly and subtly determine where and how the circulation is changing in a child.

In a clinical environment, we test circulation by timing *capillary refill*. This sounds very clever and complicated, and it is clever, but like many of these things, it is not complicated. Essentially this test times how long the capillaries, (tiny blood vessels on the surface of the skin), take to fill up from empty. The longer they take to fill, the less blood there is flowing to the extremities of the body. This can be due to a significant infection in the body, or dehydration. If capillary refill takes longer than two seconds, then that is the time to promptly involve medical professionals.

How to Test Capillary Refill

Hold the hand slightly higher than heart level and press down on the fingernail or pad of the finger until it turns white. Then let go and see how long it takes for the fingernail or pad to change colour back to pink again. It should take less than two seconds; any longer and medical intervention should be sought immediately.

Observing Fluid Intake and Output

When small children and babies are unwell, especially with a fever, their body may require more fluids than normal to remain well hydrated. Hydration simply refers to their body, their cells and their blood containing enough fluid to function properly.

Dehydration is caused by a lack of fluid in the body and poorly balanced electrolytes, meaning the body is deprived of the correct balance of liquid, salt, sugar and minerals to function properly.

Dehydration occurs when the balance between fluid consumed, (usually by food, drink or medicine), and fluid excreted (either by sweat, urine, vomit, diarrhoea and so on) is tipped in favour of excretion, so more fluid is lost from the body than is absorbed. Because babies are small they have fewer reserves of water in their bodies, which combined with immature kidneys means they can become dehydrated far more quickly and easily than a toddler or larger child. Fortunately, it is extremely easy to correct hydration levels and children recover very quickly once fluids and electrolytes are restored to their body, but prolonged dehydration can cause organ damage, organ failure and ultimately death if the signs and symptoms are not spotted and treated in a timely fashion.

Fever primarily utilises fluid in the body due to the heat it generates. Fever can also be responsible for fluid loss through sweating, through breathing more rapidly, through any vomiting or diarrhoea that may accompany a fever, or even the production of mucus from a cold. The body loses fluid continually under normal, healthy circumstances, and fever speeds up all bodily processes meaning that fluid loss is increased and happens at a more rapid rate than normal. This means that as soon as a fever appears, your child's fluid requirements will increase.

The paradox is that when a child becomes unwell, sometimes the very last thing they will want to do is to eat or drink anything. This is why small sips from small glasses are much more effective at encouraging fluid intake than being handed a large bottle or beaker. A baby who still breastfeeds is far less likely to become dehydrated because they will suckle for comfort and as a by-product of suckling, receive vital fluids. Always feed an unwell baby on demand and disregard any feeding routines you may have previously established. Any feeding routine can always be re-started once the illness has resolved itself.

Symptoms of Dehydration

- Dry mucous membranes (lips, mouth, tongue, eyes, inside of nose and so on)
- Decreased skin turgor, meaning that when skin is gently lifted between thumb and forefinger like a 'pinch', it doesn't spring back immediately when you let go
- Urine output is less than one ml/kg/hour (one millilitre of urine/per kilogram of your child's weight/per hour)

- Eyes appear sunken and dry – there are no tears
- On a baby their fontanels are sunken. Fontanels are dips or soft spaces in the skull found at the top front of the baby's head. Ask your Health Visitor, doctor or health professional to point these out to you if you are unsure where they are
- Listless and lethargic appearance
- Dry, cracked tongue

How to Assess Fluid Intake and Output (Fluid Balance)

When your child is unwell, particularly when they are less than one year old, it is extremely useful to record their *Fluid Balance*. This is usually only necessary if your child is not eating or drinking and they have an increased loss of fluids through fever, diarrhoea, vomiting, or increased effort with breathing for a sustained period of time such as four hours or more. This gives a useful insight for any medical professional as to the hydration status and requirements of your child. It is a very easy chart (see Fluid Balance Chart), to complete yourself, and whilst trying to make it as accurate as possible, don't get overly neurotic about every single millilitre. What you are trying to create with your chart is a general picture of how well hydrated your child is, or is not, as the case may be.

Measurements

Measure any fluids your child drinks in millilitres, and write down the amount of solids your child eats measured in teaspoons. An example is given on the Fluid Balance Chart for your reference. One teaspoon equates to approximately 5ml.

When measuring fluid output, for example urine, vomit, diarrhoea and so on, it helps to know how much a clean nappy, potty or vomit bowl weighs. Then when a nappy (or other vessel) has been used, you weigh everything together on normal kitchen scales in grams. Then subtract the weight of the empty nappy or container and convert the grams in weight into millilitres, which is the easiest bit, because 1g = 1ml.

Example:

   Clean nappy = 5g

   Nappy with urine and diarrhoea = 53g

   53g – 5g = 48g which equates to 48ml to record on the Fluid Balance
   chart in the Output column.

It should be quite obvious whether your child is at risk of dehydration when looking at the Fluid Balance chart. If the output is greater than input on your chart, then call and speak to your doctor or medical practitioner. If your child is passing very little urine, less than what is considered to be within normal ranges (see Fluid Balance chart and Normal Fluid/Urine Output section below for details), then this is also the time to seek medical advice and assistance. If you have any concerns you can call your GP surgery and talk to a GP or Nurse Practitioner or call 111 (in the UK) and have a discussion over the phone providing them with the figures from your chart, your child's history with this particular episode of illness, and your own intuition and observations of your child. If you are still concerned you can take your child to be assessed in person at your doctor's surgery or Emergency Department.

Food and Drink to Rehydrate

The best drinks are:

* Breast milk or formula
* Water with or without a couple of drops of fresh lemon juice added
* Herbal tea, sweetened
* Coconut water
* Clear, plain broth, stock or low-salt boullion
* The best foods are:
* Fruit – berries and soft fruit especially
* Fruit puree
* Soup/clear broth
* Ice cream
* Jelly

For your information, I have included below normal fluid requirements and normal fluid outputs for children. It will involve some basic maths if you are interested in having a comparison and knowledge of what is considered 'normal' when assessing your own child.

Normal Fluid Requirements
N.B. This includes fluid contained in food, not just liquid drinks.

To calculate normal fluid requirement per day for a normal healthy child, you will need to weigh them or know their approximate weight in kg. The following calculation is based on the recommendations made by the Advanced Life Support Group (2011).

Body Weight	Fluid Requirement Over 24 hours ml/kg
First 10kg	100ml/kg
Second 10kg	50ml/kg
Subsequent kg	20ml/kg

So, for example, if your baby weighed 8kg then their normal fluid requirements for a 24 hour period is 8kg x 100ml = 800ml of fluid required.

If your child weighed 13kg then their normal fluid requirements for a 24 hour period is;

First 10kg @ 100ml/kg (10x100) = 1000ml + Second 3kg @ 50ml/kg (3x50) = 150ml, giving a total of 1150ml of fluid required.

Normal Urine/Fluid Output

1 – 2ml/kg/hr is an average output over a period of time. You will need to take the total amount of urine passed and divide it over however many hours you have been monitoring urine output (no more than 24 hours at a time).

For example: Petra weighs 6kg. She should pass no less than 6 ml of urine per hour, (the calculation for this is 1ml/kg/hr of urine as a minimum, so Petra weighs 6kg which is 1 x 6 to calculate minimum urine output for Petra according to her weight, per hour = 6ml.) Over four hours Petra has passed 28ml urine, so to calculate her average hourly urine output 28ml urine divided by the four hour time period = 7mls of urine per hour approximately.

N.B. *You should be concerned and involve a medical professional if your child produces less than 1ml/kg/hr of urine as an average. Please see the Assessment and Observation Chart and Traffic Light System below for further guidance and information.*

The Assessment Tools

If you are anxious or need a more structured, supportive approach with clear parameters when assessing your child, then I have provided some tools and charts to help you. Even if you are confident in caring for your child, it is useful to have something to refer to in times of doubt or exhaustion when you feel like you just can't think straight.

The first tool is a simple table of what are considered 'normal' ranges for breathing, circulation, urine output and temperature. This may be enough for you to simply have this knowledge to hand. If you require more specific and detailed information, then referring to the Traffic Light System offers guidance regarding early signs and symptoms of deterioration and when you should seek further help. The Traffic Light System can be further used in conjunction with the Assessment and Observation Chart and Fluid Balance Chart. These should help you feel that you are correctly observing your child, are in control and are in a position to spot early signs of improvement or deterioration. As your experience and confidence grows, dependence on these tools should diminish. It is entirely up to you to decide which tools you need to use, and it isn't essential to use any of them. Please feel free to photocopy or download these charts from our Facebook page as and when you need them, www.facebook.com/CollaborativeHealthOfficial.

Physiological Observations Chart: Normal Ranges

Age (years)	Breathing Rate or Respiratory Rate (breaths per minute)	Capillary Refill	Urine Output	Temperature
≤1	30-40	<2 seconds	>2ml/kg/hr	36.1-37.5
1-2	25-35	<2 seconds	>1.5ml/kg/hr	36.1-37.5
2-5	25-30	<2 seconds	>1.5ml/kg/hr	36.1-37.5
5-12	20-25	<2 seconds	>1ml/kg/hr	36.1-37.5
>12	15-20	<2seconds	>1ml/kg/hr	36.1-37.5

The Traffic Light System for Identifying Risk of Serious Illness*

Green – Low RiskObserve	Amber – Medium Risk Notify or be seen by a medical professional	Red – High Risk Be seen immediately by a doctor or paramedic. Go immediately to an Emergency Department
Breathing - None of the amber or red signs	- Nostrils flaring - Breathing quickly Age 6-12 months >50 breaths per minute Age over 12 months >40 breaths per minute - Audible wheeze or 'crackles' breathing in or out - Shallow breathing	- Grunting when breathing - Breathing out heavily with pursed lips – as if blowing out a candle - Breathing quickly >60 breaths per minute - Sucking in of skin in between ribs, collar bones or base of throat when breathing in - Appears to be working hard to breathe
Circulation & Hydration - Normal colour - Capillary refill <2 Seconds - Normal skin and eyes - Moist mucus membranes	- Change in pallor - Capillary refill >2 seconds - Dry mucus membranes (lack of tears when crying, dry mouth and lips) - Poor feeding in infants - Reduced urine output, an average of less than 1ml/kg/hr	- Reduced skin turgor - Cold & clammy skin - Pale/mottled/ashen/blue in colour - Sunken fontanelle
Behaviour & Activity - Responds normally to social cues - Stays awake or awakens quickly - Strong normal cry/ not crying	- Not responding normally to social cues - No smile - Wakes only with prolonged stimulation - Decreased activity	- No response to social cues - Appears very ill - Does not wake, or if roused will not stay awake - Weak, high pitched or continuous cry
Other - None of the amber or red signs	- Age 3-6 months and fever >39 degrees Celsius - Fever > 5 days - Pain/swelling of limb or joint, or not weight bearing on a limb or using an extremity. This is an early sign of potential meningitis/sepsis	- Age 0-3 months and fever >38 degrees Celsius - Non-blanching rash - Bulging fontanelle - Neck stiffness - Seizures - Holding an odd/rigid posture when lying down or being moved

*Adapted from The Traffic Light System for Identifying Risk of Serious Illness (May 2013) National Institute of Care Excellence (NICE) Clinical Guideline 160.

Assessment and Observations Chart

Use this in conjunction with the Traffic Light System and Fluid Balance Chart to help create a 'picture' of your child's health.

BREATHING

Date	Time	Breaths per minute	Observations e.g. effort, wheezing, cough (see Traffic Light System)	Treatment given

CIRCULATION

Date	Time	Capillary refill time	Observations e.g. colour, temperature (see Traffic Light System)	Treatment given

GENERAL OBSERVATIONS

Date	Time	General observations e.g behaviour, temperature, fluids, appetite, activity, pain (see Traffic Light System)	Treatment given

Fluid Balance Chart

Date	Time	Amount of food/fluid in	Type of fluid or food	Amount of fluid out	Type of fluid out e.g. urine, vomit
TOTAL IN				TOTAL OUT	

TOTAL FLUID BALANCE _____

To calculate fluid balance, deduct TOTAL IN from TOTAL OUT and record it as either a + or − (positive if more fluid has gone in than come out, negative if more fluid has come out than gone in) in the space above that says **TOTAL FLUID BALANCE**.

For further information see How to Assess Fluid Intake and Output (fluid balance) in the chapter on Assessing Your Child.

Note 1mg = 1ml (useful when weighing nappies, vomit bowls etc.)
    1 teaspoon = 5ml (useful when feeding yoghurt or puree!)

Chapter Five

Glossary of Ingredients for Home Remedies

This chapter is an introduction to the ingredients used in the home remedies suggested in this book, which you will see in Part Two of this book. The ingredients have been chosen for their gentleness and efficacy when treating fevers and many have been used for centuries in cultures across Europe and the rest of the world. I have ensured that the ingredients are easy to obtain and there are remedies to suit every budget. Please note that the idea is not that you treat your child with every remedy suggested, but that you find the ones that you feel comfortable using, that your child is happy to have, and that fit in with your personal philosophy on health and wellbeing as well as your bank balance.

This chapter can give you the opportunity to get some of the remedies and ingredients into your home and stock up your medicine cabinet before illness strikes. If you have the time or inclination you might like to try some of the teas yourself, or even indulge in a herbal bath so you can practise making a tea or bath and also experience for yourself what it might be like for your child. This way you can have something to hand and feel prepared when your child does develop a fever, and if you are prepared then you will be less likely to panic. Well, that's the theory anyway!

Sweeteners

Honey

Since ancient times honey has been used medicinally by humans. Current medical science is finally beginning to catch up and provide evidence for the knowledge our ancestors instinctively had. In cases of fever, honey offers no immediate relief, but as a supportive medicine it has great value.

Firstly, honey is an inhibitor of bacterial and viral replication; this means that it can help limit infection of viral or bacterial origin by stopping the germs reproducing. It is also a very good energy source, as it is designed, after all, to keep bees in tiptop condition during the winter months, providing them with energy and essential nutrients.

Fever and the process of fighting infection uses a lot of energy and leaches trace vitamins and minerals from a child's body. The human body easily absorbs and utilises energy and nutrition from honey, so just a teaspoon in some herbal tea to add sweetness can provide a child who is not eating with a vital boost for their body. Honey can also support an ailing child by helping to balance electrolytes that may have been lost whilst sweating out a fever.

However, all honey is not created equally, and some can be extremely expensive. You do tend to get what you pay for. My advice would be to go for locally produced, raw honey from a reputable source if possible, and the darker the colour of the honey, the better. Honey that is dark or a rich amber colour has been cited in some studies as containing more nutrients, vitamins and antioxidants than lighter coloured honey. A local bee-keeping association is worth contacting to buy the best, and frequently best-value honey.

It is worth avoiding generic supermarket honey when using it to support a child who is unwell. Honey sold in supermarkets has often been heat-treated and processed, and sometimes diluted with sugar to reduce the costs. That is fine to have on toast every day as a condiment, but offers little value medicinally.

You may have heard of Manuka honey, which has been famously promoted for its potent medicinal properties, and this is reflected in the price. Some Manuka honey costs more than gold, weight for weight. If you are able to get hold of good quality, raw local honey then it shouldn't be necessary to spend extra on Manuka honey. When I use raw Manuka honey at home it is sparingly and generally only topically for skin infections or infections in the mouth and tonsils, not for general medicinal use, and I make sure a little goes a long, long way!

Maple Syrup

Maple syrup is similar to honey in the sense that the darker and less refined the syrup is (usually marked as Grade 2 or 'cooking grade'), the greater the mineral content compared to the paler and more refined Grade 1 Maple syrup. Also, generally speaking, Grade 2 syrup is cheaper.

Maple syrup is rich in trace minerals, especially iron and is an excellent substitute for honey, particularly if you have a child who doesn't have a sweet tooth, as it is less sickly sweet. Maple syrup is safe for use in children under one year of age, which is another advantage over honey.

Maple syrup can be quite expensive, but a little can go a long way. Beware of cheaper Maple 'flavoured' syrups, these are just flavoured sugar and offer no nutritional value to your child at all.

Other Sweeteners

There are many alternative ways to sweeten teas and food for your child whilst simultaneously offering nutrition, energy and trace minerals. A few you might like to consider are: unrefined sugar, date syrup, black strap molasses, coconut syrup or sugar, brown rice syrup, stevia or xylitol to name just a few. Please look into these yourself and try a few to see which your child prefers.

Your local health food shop can offer you great advice about natural sweeteners, so please ask them.

Herbs

Rosemary

This is an ancient herb used for centuries in both a medicinal and culinary context with an excellent safety record. In medieval texts a rosemary bath was referred to as "the bath of life" by Gervase Markham, a 16th century English poet and writer. The Romans considered rosemary a powerful herb to help rally the body and mind, strengthening and supporting them after a long day fighting or marching.

Pliny, Dioscorides, Galen and Hippocrates (all historically important figures in medicine) mention rosemary for its exceptional cure-all qualities. It was also revered by gypsies who often consumed a small sprig of rosemary in tea as a general tonic for the body and to ward off disease. In fact, rosemary tea is still the custom in parts of Italy and Greece, especially where the famous Blue-Zones are (areas known for exceptional health and longevity of the people resident there), and it is thought that consumption of rosemary tea may play a role in the extraordinary number of active and healthy centenarians there.

A rosemary bath revitalises the body helping to imbue the child with the strength to fight illness, as well as having the advantage of being an antiseptic and analgesic. Used in a herbal morning bath following a night of fever, rosemary supports recovery, increases vitality, refreshes the child generally and is a useful tonic for general aches, pains, headaches and malaise, which oftentimes accompany a fever.

Rosemary leaves are also thought to stimulate and strengthen the body after illness, and to help if exhaustion is an issue such as with viral fatigue. It is an effective and valuable herb for convalescence and recovery.

Chamomile

Chamomile is renowned for its soothing and cooling properties with regards to childhood fevers. The herbalist Parkinson wrote of chamomile, that it is,

> "...both for the sick and the sound, in bathing to comfort and strengthen the sound, and to ease pain in the diseased."

Culpeper, the famous medieval herbalist said of a chamomile bath:

> "Bathing with chamomile removes weariness and eases pain whatever part of the body it is employed."

Beatrix Potter had Mrs Rabbit give Peter Rabbit a spoonful of chamomile tea for a fever, and then put him straight to bed. Chamomile has worked for centuries, and it still prevails.

Chamomile tea is a powerful anti-inflammatory, a potent immune booster, is a proven sedative and a mild relaxant. It helps to calm an anxious child and in traditional folk medicine chamomile was viewed as a cooling herb, as it removes heat from the body and areas of inflammation. Chamomile is still used in mainland Europe as the primary herb to treat childhood fevers; indeed, in Germany pharmacies sell chamomile suppositories to treat fever in young children and babies. It is gentle and potent, complementing the action of lime flowers perfectly.

Lime Flower (Linden Flower)

Lime flowers are considered invaluable and safe for reducing childhood fevers, calming restless and hysterical children, easing tension and as an effective sleep aid. It makes a very mild and pleasant-tasting tea and is therefore easy to disguise in juice or formula. However, because it is so mild-tasting, lime flower tea is usually the easiest tea to get a child to drink *without* the need to disguise its flavour. It is a wonderful introductory tea if your child has not tried herbal tea before. Babies, children and breastfeeding mothers alike can drink it safely in large amounts.

Lime flowers can reduce a fever just enough to increase the comfort of the child without diminishing their immune response. It manages to do this by encouraging the body to sweat gently. Lime flower tea can also be used to relieve headaches, nausea and vomiting, all symptoms frequently associated with childhood fever. It is an exceptional herb at reducing catarrhal conditions, so is ideal when used for feverish colds and flu.

Lemons

Aside from being an extremely rich source of vitamin C, lemons contain a wide range of minerals perfect for replenishing lost electrolytes during a fever. A couple of drops of fresh lemon juice added to drinking water contains the antimicrobial properties of the humble lemon and will also reduce fever. The exact process by which the lemon reduces a fever is unclear, but what is clear is that it works.

Used as a topical application via Lemon Socks or Lemon Legs (please see the chapter on Practical Nursing Therapies at Home for instructions), fever is reduced and comfort levels of the child increased. The theories relating to the medicinal properties of the lemon are plentiful, but evidence, other than anecdotal and experiential, is scarce. The main reason that the lemon is considered so effective at providing comfort during a fever is explained by the nature of the plant itself. A lemon tree can withstand tremendous heat and actually thrives under these conditions. It is because of these qualities that various branches of medicine utilise the lemon to treat fever, and why it is believed to be so successful in reducing fever, or at least enabling the patient to tolerate fever better.

Treating a fever using lemons calms the child and increases comfort levels enabling the child to rest more peacefully. The fever is often reduced enough to put the parent's mind at ease within half an hour of treatment.

Lavender

Lavender is well known for being gentle in its action but powerful in its efficacy. It is strongly antibacterial, anti-fungal and antiseptic, as well as having calming and mood-lifting qualities. It is reputed to bring balance to the body, calming the circulatory system, reducing high blood pressure and soothing a rapidly beating heart. These are all aspects of a fever that can contribute to anxiety, discomfort and insomnia.

Lavender is considered to be a cooling herb for the body, dispelling excess heat. It is reputed to be restorative and purifying, which is in essence the purpose of fever, thus supporting the body in its action. It is commonly found growing in gardens, and although it makes a bitter tasting tea, its medicinal properties are easily absorbed through the skin in a bath, where the delicious aroma can also be enjoyed.

Lemon Balm

Lemon balm is gently cooling for a fever, has potent anti-viral properties and relieves anxiety and restlessness. It makes a delicious, mild-tasting tea, so is excellent for children, and the fresh herb exudes a wonderfully uplifting aroma in a bath. It is commonly found growing prolifically in gardens as it is a member of the mint family.

Lemon balm helps to dispel headaches, nausea and vomiting, which can all be experienced by children with a high fever. It also soothes the circulatory system, calms a racing heart and slows rapid breathing, bringing a sense of peace to the body without inhibiting the purpose of fever. It is uplifting and encourages a positive outlook, so quite a useful cup of tea for the parent looking after an unwell child too!

Elderflower

Elderflowers are the fragrant white blossoms that precede the dark black berries. The elder tree is quite a scruffy-looking plant, seemingly neither tree nor bush, and is frequently found in gardens, hedgerows and wasteland around the UK. It is an ancient tree, known in medieval times as 'Nature's Medicine Chest', as every part of the tree was utilised for curing a wide range of ailments.

The tree is surrounded by myth and legend, and there is no denying the health-giving properties of the elder. Modern science is finally vindicating what the Native Americans and Wise Women of ancient times have known all along. The flowers are especially potent at reducing fever, and are mild-tasting in a tea or tincture. A strong elderflower syrup or cordial may also impart similar benefits, although perhaps is not as potent as the tea.

The flowers reduce inflammation and dispel heat in the body. They are also very effective at relieving catarrhal congestion, so this tea has earned its reputation for treating influenza, bronchitis and any number of conditions where fever and catarrh are a tandem issue. In our house, we combine elderflowers with either lime flowers or lemon balm as a potent anti-viral, fever busting, catarrh clearing, anti-inflammatory, powerhouse of a tea.

Elderberry

Elderberries have been studied extensively by conventional science and have been found to contain, amongst its many health benefits and immune-boosting properties, good levels of vitamin A and extremely high levels of vitamin C, B6 and iron. Elderberries have also been shown to be extremely effective at combatting the flu virus and reducing the severity and duration of infection.

However, it is the fever-reducing capabilities of the elderberry that we are most interested in for the purpose of this book. Elderberries are extremely effective at removing heat from the body. They can be taken internally for fever or used as a poultice externally on joints or wounds that are exuding heat, inflammation and redness. Coupled with this cooling ability are the powerful anti-viral properties of the berries combined with vitamins and minerals known to support the body when fighting infection.

The elder is a sacred plant to Native American Indians and they have used the berries for centuries as a general immune tonic as well as to reduce inflammation, remove heat from infections, and lower fevers. Typically, they would crush berries in honey to take as a medicine internally for fevers, and I think that elderberries taken this way or as a syrup, is one of the most delicious medicines known to man!

Aside from elderberries having proven and potent anti-viral properties, this is a tree also surrounded with European Wise Woman myth and ancient folklore. It is said that an old crone lives in the elder tree, and this wise old crone wants nothing more than to have her tree used as medicine. But the old crone in the elder does not tolerate disrespect, and so traditionally, before harvesting, the men or women would ask the tree for permission to use her berries, bark or flowers and request that the crone imbue them with healing powers. Once this ancient ritual was completed, they were free to harvest with her permission and blessing!

Thyme

This is my favourite herb. Thyme is powerful, yet gentle enough to earn an excellent reputation as a children's herb. In Germany and Austria, thyme is frequently found as an ingredient in herbal remedies for children. Indeed, the Abbess Hildegard of Bingen was a huge fan of Thyme. Hildegard was an intellectual and polymath who lived in the 11th century in Germany. She is considered to have invented the study of natural science as well as writing some of the first medical textbooks citing botanical studies that she herself had conducted. A formidable woman, when it was a difficult time to be formidable and also a woman, Hildegard was a passionate advocate of thyme for many illnesses as well as a general immune tonic. She observed,

"He who drinks a cup of thyme tea in the morning will soon feel the beneficial effect: enlivened spirits, great comfort in the stomach, no coughing in the morning and an overall well-being."

In terms of thyme specifically treating fever, it is more of a wholistic addition to a bath. It supports the actions of other herbs, and the unwell child in general terms. Thyme is known to ease nervousness and anxiety, aid relaxation and restful sleep, support the body in the elimination of waste and support the immune system generally. It also has potent antibacterial, anti-inflammatory and anti-viral properties.

Rudolph Steiner, the founder of Anthroposophical Medicine, also advocates the use of thyme for children. His teachings are instrumental in inspiring the ingredients for the Weleda Baby and Child Calendula Bath, which is recommended later in this book. Steiner considered Thyme to be a herb which replenishes a child's energy and he believed that regular thyme baths strengthen children physically, immunologically and emotionally.

Echinacea

I would love to include the incredible herb echinacea in this book on fever, and recommend its use to you in the form of a tincture or glycerite. However, I am writing this in Britain where we are restricted from using or advising its use in children under the age of twelve years old. This law came to pass due to a very small number (single figures) of allergic reactions in young children. Given the number of allergic reactions children have to many common, everyday ingestibles, such as milk, peanuts, pine nuts, strawberries and so on, none of these which have limitations placed on them by law, the law applying to echinacea seems a bit extreme and overly cautious. This is especially true when you consider this herb has been used for centuries by native and indigenous populations and has an outstanding safety record.

Other countries (at the time of writing this book) do not have this same recommendation or law limiting the use of echinacea, notably New Zealand and currently also America and Australia. I have used several products containing echinacea for my children since they were babies, which I mention later in the book. My advice would be to research echinacea yourself, and to talk to a qualified Medical Herbalist or Herbal Pharmacist or Apothecary. They are allowed to prescribe echinacea for any age in an appropriate form and dosage and are well-trained in possible side effects, risks and contraindications. I have yet to meet a herbalist who agrees with restricting echinacea to children over 12 years old, but you may encounter one!

Susun S. Weed, a very experienced wise woman and herbalist, recommends echinacea for treating fever in infants in her book, *The Wise Woman Herbal for the Child Bearing Year.* She also advocates breastfeeding mothers taking echinacea themselves in order to pass it on to their baby via breastmilk.

Incidentally, there are no restrictions preventing children drinking echinacea in the form of tea or making your own glycerites and tinctures for personal and family use, (see the Resources section for suggestions of some of the many books available instructing on making home remedies).

Essential Oils

Rosemary

Historically Greeks and Romans saw rosemary as a symbol of regeneration, and French hospitals used to burn rosemary during epidemics to cleanse the air. Both the regenerative and disinfecting powers of the herb are amongst the reasons the essential oil is recommended to treat fever.

Rosemary essential oil is seen as a cooling oil on the one hand, and yet able to relieve chilliness and shivering from cold on the other. It has a refreshing fragrance that clears the mind and revives the senses, and pain-relieving qualities that can soothe muscular aches as well as headaches. In essence, this oil is wonderful for treating the symptoms of fever and the aches and malaise that accompany fever.

It is recommended for use in the morning or during the day, as it is a stimulating oil. It revives and increases the sense of vitality, enlivening the body in the process. After an exhausting night of fever, rosemary oil will lift and refresh the mind and body of the child. Because of the stimulating nature of the essential oil, it should be avoided during pregnancy and if suffering from epilepsy. Using the herb itself, rather than the essential oil, is a milder form of administering the medicinal properties of this remarkable herb.

Bergamot

Bergamot is known for its cooling properties both physically by reducing fever, and emotionally by taking the heat out of anger. It is a delicate oil with a slight citrus scent that is gentle and effective. It is native to Italy where it has been used for centuries in traditional medicine.

Bergamot nourishes, soothes and lifts the spirit and is renowned for treating anxious and depressive states. It has antibiotic properties, as well as a proven reputation for combatting viral and fungal infections. It is thought to assist in cleansing as well as cooling the body as it gently encourages sweating. It soothes aches and pains and prepares the body for rest and recuperation.

Combined with the potent immune boosting qualities of thyme, a peaceful night is hopefully encouraged and assured.

Thyme Linalol

Not to be confused with thyme vulgaris, which is a much stronger essential oil and can cause skin irritation if used topically, thyme linalol (sweet thyme), is a more suitable and gentle essential oil for use with children. It doesn't irritate the skin so can be applied topically as long as it is diluted, used as an inhalation or added to a bath.

Thyme is an ancient herb that has been used for both medicinal and culinary purposes to great effect for centuries. It was traditionally thought that, just by carrying a sprig of thyme, you could evoke courage and ensure protection from infection. The Ancient Egyptians used thyme as part of the embalming process, and Hildegard of Bingen used thyme as her primary herb in the treatment of leprosy with excellent results.

Thyme is a potent immune tonic and promotes the production of white blood cells to assist the body in fighting infection. It also prevents the spread of germs as it is a powerful antimicrobial oil. It soothes aches and pains, lifts low spirits and combats feelings of exhaustion. A bath with a couple of drops of thyme linalol offers a generally supportive role for treating fever.

Lemon Oil

Lemon oil has a refreshing and sunny aroma, it is difficult not to feel better just catching a whiff of it! Fortunately, it also has some very useful properties when it comes to treating fever in children. Along with Thyme, this oil is said to stimulate the production of white blood cells and invigorate them so they boost immune function. It is also very effective at reducing high temperatures, and acts as a general tonic, purifying the body generally.

Lemon oil is naturally antiseptic and a potent antiviral, and is said to ease anaemia, headaches and general aches and pains. It is a cooling oil which is soothing to the body and mind, perfect to use before bed ensuring comfort for the night and encouraging rest.

In Conclusion

Our state of health is a very personal journey, fluctuating throughout our lives and meaning different things to different people. How we support our children through illness and encourage a healthy immune response to disease can help build their resilience as they go into adulthood.

We are heading towards a time when effective antibiotics will be hard to come by and our leading doctors and scientists are preparing for what they refer to as the *post-antibiotic apocalyptic era*. It sounds terrifying, doesn't it? In the UK, we also have an NHS at crisis point, limited and ever-diminishing resources for healthcare and a concerted push towards encouraging self-care within the community. How ironic that we are pushing people towards self-care, having encouraged dependence on pharmaceuticals and the need for pill-popping for so many years!

Mistrust in the innate and miraculous ability for the human body to heal itself has been cultivated for decades, beginning in earnest with the discovery of antibiotics. Given the miraculous nature of antibiotics, this is understandable; however, even the simplest coughs and colds have been subject to medication as an increasingly fearful and sceptical public doubted the human body's ability to recover without medical intervention and support. As time has moved on, it has become apparent that modern medicine has some, but not all, of the answers. The medical establishment is trying to gently encourage us towards greater self-reliance. And the medical establishment is right. There are times when we need medical intervention, but most often we are able to care for each other and ourselves in the comfort of our own home. It just requires a mind shift, information, simple and effective remedies and parameters to work from. My hope is that this book, and the ones that follow, will provide these for you.

Health is defined by more than just the physical and pharmaceutical. It comprises the spiritual, emotional and environmental too. Good nutrition, loving and supportive relationships, fresh air and exercise all contribute towards the overall health of a child, which in turn helps determine the resilience a child has to disease and their speedy and uncomplicated recovery when they do get unwell.

My primary intention for this book is to share information with parents who may be looking for a more natural way to support their child's health. If I have done my job well, then I also hope you feel calmer and more confident when nursing your child through a fever at home. Part Two of this book, which follows next, covers the practical hands-on treatments such as remedies, nursing therapies and recipes. Use it as a reference book, it is broken down into age-specific sections which will hopefully make it easier for you to find what you are looking for.

Part Two

Part Two

Chapter Six

Age Appropriate Treatments for Fever

Fever in Age 0-6 months old

N.B. Please consult the chapter on Assessing Your Child and the Traffic Light System for fevers in conjunction with this chapter.

If your baby develops a fever at this age I would have them assessed by a medical professional. Fever in children less than three months of age is quite uncommon and can be a sign of a serious infection.

Signs and Symptoms Your Baby May Have a Fever

- Feels hot to touch
- Has a faster breathing rate
- Has flushed cheeks
- Has an increased heart rate
- Is difficult to settle, is grisly, crying easily and difficult to comfort
- Is sleepy, difficult to wake and to keep awake
- Is feeding more frequently or less frequently
- Is nauseous and/or vomiting
- Has a raised temperature according to the thermometer, (use a digital thermometer in the armpit for children this age or a temporal artery thermometer which consists of a wand you sweep and hold over the temple area.)

Practical Tips

Remove excess clothing like socks, hats, blankets and jumpers. Babies cannot control their own body temperature at this stage in their life, so can easily get a 'fever' just by simple over-dressing and over-heating. Once the baby has had a chance to cool down, observe signs to see if the baby still has a raised temperature.

If a baby does have a fever because of being unwell, and has been seen by a doctor, then keep the baby dressed in a nappy and vest as a minimum, covered with a cotton sheet or summer sleeping bag, and in a room ideally between 18-20 degrees. Of course, you will need to use common sense with this advice depending on the ambient heat in the room, the time of year and if the baby appears too hot or is shivering because their body is trying to generate heat and increase their body temperature.

I would advocate frequent, on demand breastfeeding, or bottle (whichever is currently being used) to ensure the baby remains well hydrated (dehydration can cause a fever in a baby), and plenty of skin-to-skin cuddles with Mummy and Daddy. Nature is an extraordinary helper, and in young babies when they are cuddled skin-to-skin, (where the baby is naked, or wearing just a nappy, and the parent holds the baby against their bare chest), then the baby is automatically calmed and the parent's skin temperature will change according to the needs of the baby. So, if a baby feels too hot with fever, then the bare skin of the parent will feel cool to touch. Likewise, when the baby feels cold, then the skin of the parent will feel warm to touch. Sounds crazy? Try it and see – you will be amazed.

Aim to create a calm, quiet, peaceful environment and, in an ideal world, have someone to look after the mother or main person caring for such a young baby. The main carer will need to be well-fed, hydrated and have an opportunity for rest, because caring for such a young and unwell baby without someone in turn caring for you, is very difficult indeed. Involve fathers, grandparents, neighbours and friends to help wherever possible in this instance.

Homoeopathic Remedies
(See *Administering Homeopathic Medicines*)

Aconite 6C or 30C The first remedy to go to for sudden onset of symptoms

0–6 Months of Age

and in the early stages of a fever. The child may feel cold and suffer chills as their body tries to create a fever. The child may not want to be uncovered or undressed because they will feel the cold acutely and shiver. The child will be thirsty and restless.

Belladonna 6C or 30C A common remedy usually given once a fever is established. The characteristics are for unusual restlessness and agitation, particularly at night, and a red, flushed face. Heat is also a distinguishing factor; the head especially feels very hot to touch, with heat almost radiating off the body. In contrast hands and feet can feel cool. Delirium with fever at night is also a feature that would suggest this remedy.

Arsenicum 6C or 30C A child needing Arsenicum will feel chilly and better for being kept warm. They will be restless, anxious and thirsty for small, frequent drinks. Symptoms are usually at their worst between midnight and 2-3am.

Bryonia 6C or 30C A child needing this remedy would have the heat of fever but with an accompanying dryness of the skin and mucous membranes. A dry mouth and lips are accompanied by a thirst where the child gulps down fluid greedily. Even tiny movements cause the child to cry out in distress.

Pulsatilla 6C or 30C A child needing Pulsatilla will be weepy and need to be soothed by company or being carried and rocked continually. They will want to sleep with the parent and be quite clingy and whiny. A Pulsatilla child will not be thirsty at all and feel much better in the open air, or with access to fresh air. It is especially important that a child needing Pulsatilla is prevented from getting a chill when exposed to fresh air.

Chamomilla 6C or 30C The child is irritable and restless, almost appearing angry or in pain. They may be screaming and crying, feeling hot even on their extremities. They may have hot feet especially, which they don't want covered and will kick covers off. They can't abide heat, or being cold or fresh air; nothing is right and the child is inconsolable unless being carried or rocked. The parent or carer will often feel at a total loss and as if they can't do a thing right for the child.

Nux Vomica 6C or 30C A child needing Nux Vomica has frequently developed a fever as a result of a change in diet, eating rich foods, or lack of sleep. In a young baby, it can be a change from breast milk to formula, or being around a lot of family and being passed from one relative to another. For an older child, it is the classic remedy to give for a fever after a birthday party with lots of excitement, sugary food and drinks. Frequently digestive issues such as diarrhoea or constipation and headaches accompany a fever. The child will feel chilly and want to be covered at all times.

Ferrum Phos. Bio Chemic Tissue Salt This is a good remedy for the early stages of a fever and is the classic remedy for inflammation and slow onset of fever. This is the remedy for fevers with few obvious causes or symptoms. Ferrum Phos is often indicated for fevers that occur after a period of over-exertion, or when a child seems off colour, not quite themselves but with no obvious cause. It is often a useful remedy in recuperation where the child feels tired easily and is generally low in energy.

Combination Homeopathic Remedies

ABC Remedy – This is a simple combination remedy comprising Aconite, Belladonna and Chamomilla, either in 30C or 6C potency. Most homeopathic pharmacies make a version of this. It is available from both Weleda and Helios and can be ordered on their websites. Good local Health Food shops and pharmacies such as Boots may also stock this remedy. If you can't get hold of it you can dissolve one homeopathic pillule each of Aconite, Belladonna and Chamomilla into some water and give small sips to your child, either from a bottle, with a medicinal dropper or syringe, or a small cup.

This is a great remedy for children with non-specific symptoms and in the early stages of fever. It is extremely effective for teething-related symptoms too when the child is grisly, clingy, fussy and has red cheeks and sore gums and a mild fever. It is a wonderful go-to, catch-all remedy for the busy or confused parent and amateur homeopath alike and is often the first remedy given in our household.

Herbal Remedies

Herbal Baths

Rosemary bath in the **morning** – Using either one large handful of fresh rosemary or one tablespoon of dried rosemary or three teabags of rosemary tea, and follow the instructions on Herbal Baths in the chapter How to Use the Remedies in this Book.

While the baby is in the bath, gently bathe the body of the baby with the herbal tea bath using a flannel or your cupped hands. Don't wet the baby's hair though if the baby has a temperature or is unwell.

A rosemary bath is refreshing and revitalising for a baby, and using fresh or dried herbs rather than essential oils is a very gentle way of giving a child the therapeutic benefits of the herb.

Remove the baby from the bath after 15 minutes or when the baby has had enough, gently wrap the child in a towel and pat dry. Dress in appropriate fresh clothes for the day.

Chamomile tea bath in the **evening** – Using either two handfuls of dried chamomile flowers, or four chamomile tea bags, and follow the instructions on Herbal Baths in the chapter How to Use the Remedies in this Book.

Follow the same bathing routine as explained for the morning rosemary bath above. Chamomile is gentle and soothing for a baby, and will help ensure a restful night.

Remove the baby from the bath and gently pat dry with a towel. Put the baby into fresh nightclothes ready for bed. Use Lemon Legs therapy (described later in this chapter) if your baby still needs some help to settle for the night.

Herbal Tea

Please follow the instructions on Making a Herbal Tea in the chapter How to Use the Remedies in this Book. These are two very mild tasting herbal teas, and traditionally very safe and easy to persuade children to take.

Lime Flower (sometimes known as Linden Flower) tea – This is the milder-tasting out of the two teas suggested here. Allow the flowers to infuse for 15 minutes and then remove the herbs. Try to give a teaspoon or two of the herbal tea (5-10mls) every three hours for up to four doses, (20-40mls) per 12 hour period.

Once sufficiently cooled, the tea can be sipped day and night.

Chamomile tea – This can either be given on its own or combined with the lime flower tea. Allow to brew for 15 minutes. Administer a teaspoon or two of the herbal tea (5-10mls) every three hours for up to four doses, (20-40mls) per 12 hour period.

The tea can be sipped day and night.

If you don't want to combine the herbs together then you can always alternate them, giving one teaspoon of lime flower tea followed by a teaspoon of chamomile tea, and so on.

Other Remedies and Treatments

Lemon Legs
(See chapter on *Practical Nursing Therapies at Home for instructions*)

This is a variation on the Lemon Socks therapy that is suggested later in the book. The reason for this variation is that it is considered poor practice in some fields of medicine to cool the feet of a young baby, let alone allow the feet to be wet. In contrast, reflexologists consider the foot to reflect and map the whole body, in which case cooling the feet actually can be seen as cooling the entire body. So, the jury is out, but I personally prefer this method for babies where the feet are left and the lower legs are wrapped instead. I first saw this therapy used in a children's hospital in India to great effect.

This therapy can be used during the day, but I think it works best after a bedtime bath when putting the baby to bed. The treatment helps to reduce a fever slightly and enable a restful sleep. If the baby wakes in the night with a high fever and is restless and uncomfortable, then simply refresh the compress in the lemon water and apply again to the legs.

For sensitive or broken skin, you can create a compress the same way but using cooled tea from lime flowers or chamomile as a substitute for lemon juice or vinegar. You won't need to dilute the tea, just add 500-800mls of freshly boiled water to two to three teabags, or three teaspoons of loose herbal tea and allow the tea to brew for 20-30 minutes and then cool to body temperature. Then soak the muslin or cotton wool in the tea, wring out excess water and apply to the calves of the baby and cover with leggings to hold compress in place.

Lemon is cooling for children who have a fever. Using lemon in a damp compress also encourages cooling of the baby through gentle evaporation and heat exchange. When a baby has a fever, you can find that within an hour or so the compress is virtually dry. The compress can be refreshed as many times as required.

Fever in Age 6-12 months old

N.B. Please consult the chapter on Assessing Your Child and the Traffic Light System for fevers in conjunction with this chapter.

If you are ever concerned about a fever in your baby, I would always advise consulting a medical professional. Once your baby has been seen and a diagnosis given, you can proceed how you wish in terms of supporting your child through illness.

Signs and Symptoms Your Baby May Have a Fever

- Feels hot to touch
- Has a faster breathing rate
- Has flushed cheeks
- Has an increased heart rate
- Is difficult to settle, is grisly, crying easily and difficult to comfort
- Is sleepy, difficult to wake and to keep awake
- Is feeding more frequently or less frequently
- Rejects food offered
- Is nauseous and/or vomiting
- The child has a raised temperature according to the thermometer. You can use a digital thermometer in the armpit for children this age or a temporal artery thermometer, which consists of a wand you sweep and hold over the temple area. A tympanic thermometer (ear thermometer) can also be used from this age, but it may be difficult to get an accurate temperature reading. I would advise taking the temperature in both ears to begin with until your confidence builds

Practical Tips

Remove excess clothing like socks, hats, blankets and cardigans or jumpers. Keep vests and nappies on though and make sure your baby doesn't get chilled in the process. Babies can still struggle to control their own body temperature at this stage in their life, so can easily get a 'fever' just by simple over-dressing and over-heating. Once your baby has had a chance to cool down, observe signs to see if your baby still has a raised temperature.

I would advocate frequent, on demand breastfeeding, or bottle (whichever is currently being used) to ensure the baby remains well hydrated (dehydration can cause a fever in a baby). If your baby is eating solids, then making simple fruit purees can encourage fluid intake. Please see Recipes for Illness for some ideas.

Try to create a calm, quiet and peaceful environment and, in an ideal world, someone to look after the mother or main person caring for your young baby. The main carer will need to be well fed, hydrated and have an opportunity for rest, because caring for a young and unwell baby without someone in turn caring for you, is very difficult indeed. Involve fathers, grandparents, neighbours and friends to help wherever possible.

Plenty of cuddles with Mummy and/or Daddy, skin-to-skin where possible to lower a fever in a baby is also still recommended (see Fever in Age 0-6 Months Old). Ensure that neither the baby nor parent gets chilled in the process though.

Homoeopathic Remedies
(See *Administering Homeopathic Medicines*)

Aconite 6C or 30C The first remedy to go to for sudden onset of symptoms and in the early stages of a fever. The child may feel cold and suffer chills as their body tries to create a fever. The child may not want to be uncovered or undressed because they will feel the cold acutely and shiver. The child will be thirsty and restless.

Belladonna 6C or 30C A common remedy usually given once a fever is established. The characteristics are for unusual restlessness and agitation, particularly at night, and a red, flushed face. Heat is also a distinguishing factor; the head especially feels very hot to touch, with heat almost radiating off the body. In contrast hands and feet can feel cool. Delirium with fever at night is also a feature that would suggest this remedy.

Arsenicum 6C or 30C A child needing Arsenicum will feel chilly and better for being kept warm. They will be restless, anxious and thirsty for small, frequent drinks. Symptoms are usually at their worst between midnight and 2-3am.

Bryonia 6C or 30C A child needing this remedy would have the heat of fever but with an accompanying dryness of the skin and mucous membranes. A dry mouth and lips are accompanied by a thirst where the child gulps down fluid greedily. Even tiny movements cause the child to cry out in distress.

Pulsatilla 6C or 30C A child needing Pulsatilla will be weepy and need to be soothed by company or being carried and rocked continually. They will want to sleep with the parent and be quite clingy and whiny. A Pulsatilla child will not be thirsty at all and feel much better in the open air, or with access to fresh air. It is especially important that a child needing Pulsatilla is prevented from getting a chill when exposed to fresh air.

Chamomilla 6C or 30C The child is irritable and restless, almost appearing angry or in pain. They may be screaming and crying, feeling hot even on their extremities. They may have hot feet especially, which they don't want covered and will kick covers off. They can't abide heat, or being cold or fresh air; nothing is right and the child is inconsolable unless being carried or rocked. The parent or carer will often feel at a total loss and as if they can't do a thing right for the child.

Nux Vomica 6C or 30C A child needing Nux Vomica has frequently developed a fever as a result of a change in diet, eating rich foods, or lack of sleep. In a young baby, it can be a change from breast milk to formula, or being around a lot of family and being passed from one relative to another. For an older child, it is the classic remedy to give for a fever after a birthday party with lots of excitement, sugary food and drinks. Frequently, digestive issues such as diarrhoea or constipation and headaches accompany a fever. The child will feel chilly and want to be covered at all times.

Ferrum Phos. Bio Chemic Tissue Salt This is a good remedy for the early stages of a fever and is the classic remedy for inflammation and slow onset of fever. This is the remedy for fevers with few obvious causes or symptoms. Ferrum Phos is often indicated for fevers that occur after a period of over-exertion, or when a child seems off colour, not quite themselves but with no obvious cause. It is often a useful remedy in recuperation where the child feels tired easily and is generally low in energy.

6–12 Months of Age

Combination Homeopathic Remedies

ABC Remedy – This is a simple combination remedy comprising Aconite, Belladonna and Chamomilla, either in 30C or 6C potency. Most homeopathic pharmacies make a version of this. It is available from both Weleda and Helios and can be ordered on their websites. Good local health food shops and pharmacies such as Boots may also stock this remedy. If you can't get hold of it you can dissolve one homeopathic pillule each of Aconite, Belladonna and Chamomilla into some water and give small sips to your child, either from a bottle, with a medicinal dropper or syringe, or a small cup.

This is a great remedy for children with non-specific symptoms and in the early stages of fever. It is extremely effective for teething-related symptoms too when the child is grisly, clingy, fussy and has red cheeks and sore gums and a mild fever. It is a wonderful go-to, catch-all remedy for the busy or confused parent and amateur homeopath alike and is often the first remedy given in our household.

Herbal Remedies

Herbal Baths

N.B. Baths suggested from the earlier section are also appropriate and useful for this age group, too.

To make a herbal bath, please follow the instructions on Herbal Baths in the chapter How to Use the Remedies in this Book.

*Rosemary, Lavender and Lemon Balm tea bath in the **morning*** – Use one large handful each of fresh rosemary, fresh lavender and fresh lemon balm. Check your garden, many of you will have these herbs and may not have realised it! Or use one tablespoon each of dried rosemary and dried lemon balm and two tablespoons of dried lavender flowers.

This herbal bath is cooling and refreshing for a baby, and using herbs rather than essential oils is a very gentle way of giving a child the therapeutic benefits of these plants.

Remove the baby from the bath after 15 minutes or when the baby has had enough. Gently wrap the child in a towel and pat dry. Dress in appropriate fresh clothes for the day.

Chamomile tea bath in the **evening** – Use either two handfuls of dried chamomile flowers, or four chamomile tea bags in your brew.

Follow the same bathing routine as explained for the morning Rosemary bath above. Chamomile is gentle and soothing for a baby, and will help ensure a restful night.

Remove the baby from the bath and gently pat dry with a towel. Put the baby into fresh nightclothes ready for bed. Use Lemon Socks therapy (as described in the chapter Practical Nursing Therapies at Home), if your baby still needs some help to settle for the night.

Herbal Tea

Please follow the instructions on Making a Herbal Tea in the chapter How to Use the Remedies in this Book. These are very mild-tasting herbal teas, and traditionally very safe and easy to persuade children to take.

Lime Flower (also known as Linden Flower) tea – Allow the flowers to infuse for 15 minutes and then remove the herbs. Try to give two to three teaspoons of the herbal tea (10-15mls) every three hours for up to four doses, (40-60mls) per 12 hour period.

The tea can also be sweetened by adding it to fruit juice or a small amount of maple syrup and can be sipped day and night.

Chamomile tea – This can either be given on its own or combined with the lime flower tea. Allow the chamomile (or chamomile and lime flower combination), to brew for 15 minutes and then remove the herbs from the boiled water.

Try to give two to three teaspoons of the herbal tea (10-15mls) every three hours for up to four doses, (40-60mls) per 12 hour period.

The tea can also be sweetened by adding it to fruit juice or a small amount of maple syrup and can be sipped day and night.

Elderflower tea – This tea can be used alone or combined for an especially wonderful tonic with both lime flower and chamomile. To brew as a single, (or combination) flower infusion, allow the herb/s to infuse for 10-15 minutes in freshly boiled water.

Try to give two to three teaspoons of the herbal tea (10-15mls) every three hours for up to four doses, (40-60mls) per 12 hour period.

If you don't want to combine the herbs together then you can always alternate the herbs, giving one teaspoon of lime flower tea followed by a teaspoon of chamomile tea, and so on.

Herbal Syrup

Elderberry (Sambucus Nigra) syrup – This panacea can be bought ready-made from health food shops, but it's easy to make yourself. However, if you do decide to buy elderberry syrup, be aware that many commercially-made syrups contain honey or additional herbs that are not recommended for children under one year of age.

There is a British company in Oxfordshire who make a wonderful elderberry syrup using just elderberry, sugar and spring water. It is delicious and I highly recommend having a look at their website where you can order it http://www.dolrosacanina.co.uk. The recipe for making your own elderberry syrup can be found in the Remedy Recipes section of this book. It is very simple and also consists only of elderberries, water and sugar.

Medical herbalists usually have elderberry syrup available to buy suitable for babies of six months and over, as would herbal apothecaries or pharmacies, which you can visit or order from online. If you have concerns then please speak to a reputed herbal pharmacy such as Botanica Medica (see Resources section) for free advice, or ask your local medical herbalist. Your local Health Food shop may also have useful advice, or consult your healthcare practitioner.

If you would like to try and make your own syrup, it is advisable to make as large a quantity of syrup as possible to see your family through the winter. A bottle of homemade elderberry syrup also makes a lovely, comforting gift for any friends, family or neighbours who are under the weather and need a pep up.

Dosage for Homemade Elderberry Syrup
One quarter teaspoon (1.25mls) mixed with a small amount of water, or added

to formula, yoghurt, porridge, fruit purees etc. to be taken up to twice per day during acute illness and fever, usually for a maximum of seven days.

Other Remedies and Treatments

Lemon Socks
(See chapter on *Practical Nursing Therapies at Home for instructions*)

This therapy can be used during the day, but it is used to best effect after a bedtime bath when putting the baby to bed.

Lemon is cooling for children who have a fever, and this is a comforting treatment for the child, and a nurturing one for the parent to give. Remember the aim is not to reduce the fever to a more acceptable level, it is to increase the comfort of the child to enable rest. This treatment will usually reduce a fever by a small amount, and it will calm and soothe the child.

Only use the lemon treatment if the child is having difficulty with the fever, i.e. showing signs of restlessness, discomfort, exhaustion or if they are feeling very hot indeed. When a baby has a fever, you can find that within 30 minutes to an hour or so the compress is virtually dry. The compress can be refreshed as many times as required.

For sensitive or broken skin, you can create this treatment the same way but using cooled tea from lime (linden) flowers or chamomile as a substitute for lemon juice or vinegar. You won't need to dilute the tea, just add 800mls of freshly boiled water to two to three teabags, or three teaspoons of loose herbal tea and allow to brew for 20-30 minutes and allow the tea to cool to body temperature. Then soak the socks in the tea, wring out excess water and apply to the feet following the instructions for the lemon socks.

Fever in Age 12 months to 3 years old

N.B. Please consult the chapter on Assessing Your Child and the Traffic Light System for fevers in conjunction with this chapter.

If you are ever concerned about a fever in your child, I would always advise consulting a medical professional. Once your child has been seen and a diagnosis given, you can proceed how you wish in terms of supporting your child through illness.

Signs and Symptoms Your Child May Have a Fever

- Feels hot to touch
- Has a faster breathing rate
- Has flushed cheeks
- Has an increased heart rate
- Is difficult to settle, is grisly, crying easily and difficult to comfort
- Is sleepy, difficult to wake and to keep awake
- Is feeding more frequently or less frequently
- Rejects food offered
- Is nauseous and/or vomiting
- Complains of feeling cold or hot
- Is clingy
- The child has a raised temperature according to the thermometer. A tympanic (ear) thermometer can be used from this age. I would advise taking the temperature in both ears to begin with until your confidence builds.

Practical Tips

You will need to use common sense regarding the clothing of your child, depending on the ambient heat in the room, the time of year and if the child appears too hot or is shivering because their body is trying to generate heat and increase their temperature.

I would support frequent, on demand breastfeeding, or bottle (if either are still being used to nourish the child) to ensure the child remains well hydrated.

12 Months to 3 Years of Age

Regular sips of sweetened herbal teas will also support hydration and provide gentle medicine to support your child's recovery. If your child is eating solids, then making simple fruit purees and jellies can encourage fluid intake. Please see Recipes for Illness for some ideas.

Try to maintain a calm, quiet and peaceful environment and, in an ideal world, someone to help support the mother or main person caring for the child. Plenty of cuddles for the child with Mummy and/or Daddy is always comforting for the child, as some children can get quite anxious when they feel unwell.

Homoeopathic Remedies
(See *Administering Homeopathic Medicines*)

Aconite 6C or 30C The first remedy to go to for sudden onset of symptoms and in the early stages of a fever. The child may feel cold and suffer chills as their body tries to create a fever. The child may not want to be uncovered or undressed because they will feel the cold acutely and shiver. The child will be thirsty and restless.

Belladonna 6C or 30C A common remedy usually given once a fever is established. The characteristics are for unusual restlessness and agitation, particularly at night, and a red, flushed face. Heat is also a distinguishing factor; the head especially feels very hot to touch, with heat almost radiating off the body. In contrast hands and feet can feel cool. Delirium with fever at night is also a feature that would suggest this remedy.

Arsenicum 6C or 30C A child needing Arsenicum will feel chilly and better for being kept warm. They will be restless, anxious and thirsty for small, frequent drinks. Symptoms are usually at their worst between midnight and 2-3am.

Bryonia 6C or 30C A child needing this remedy would have the heat of fever but with an accompanying dryness of the skin and mucous membranes. A dry mouth and lips are accompanied by a thirst where the child gulps down fluid greedily. Even tiny movements cause the child to cry out in distress.

Pulsatilla 6C or 30C A child needing Pulsatilla will be weepy and need to be soothed by company or being carried and rocked continually. They will want to sleep with the parent and be quite clingy and whiny. A Pulsatilla child will not be thirsty at all and feel much better in the open air, or with access to fresh air. It is especially important that a child needing Pulsatilla is prevented from getting a chill when exposed to fresh air.

Chamomilla 6C or 30C The child is irritable and restless, almost appearing angry or in pain. They may be screaming and crying, feeling hot even on their extremities. They may have hot feet especially, which they don't want covered and will kick covers off. They can't abide heat, or being cold or fresh air; nothing is right and the child is inconsolable unless being carried or rocked. The parent or carer will often feel at a total loss and as if they can't do a thing right for the child.

Nux Vomica 6C or 30C A child needing Nux Vomica has frequently developed a fever as a result of a change in diet, eating rich foods, or lack of sleep. In a young baby, it can be a change from breast milk to formula, or being around a lot of family and being passed from one relative to another. For an older child, it is the classic remedy to give for a fever after a birthday party with lots of excitement, sugary food and drinks. Frequently digestive issues such as diarrhoea or constipation and headaches accompany a fever. The child will feel chilly and want to be covered at all times.

Ferrum Phos. Bio Chemic Tissue Salt This is a good remedy for the early stages of a fever and is the classic remedy for inflammation and slow onset of fever. This is the remedy for fevers with few obvious causes or symptoms. Ferrum Phos is often indicated for fevers that occur after a period of over-exertion, or when a child seems off colour, not quite themselves but with no obvious cause. It is often a useful remedy in recuperation where the child feels tired easily and is generally low in energy.

Combination Homeopathic Remedies

ABC Remedy – This is a simple combination remedy comprising Aconite, Belladonna and Chamomilla, either in 30C or 6C potency. Most homeopathic pharmacies make a version of this. It is available from both Weleda and Helios and can be ordered on their websites. Good local Health Food shops and pharmacies such as Boots may also stock this remedy. If you can't get hold of it you can dissolve one homeopathic pillule each of Aconite, Belladonna and Chamomilla into some water and give small sips to your child, either from a bottle, with a medicinal dropper or syringe, or a small cup.

This is a great remedy for children with non-specific symptoms and in the early stages of fever. It is extremely effective for teething-related symptoms too when the child is grisly, clingy, fussy and has red cheeks and sore gums and a mild fever. It is a wonderful go-to, catch-all remedy for the busy or confused parent and amateur homeopath alike and is often the first remedy given in our household.

Herbal Remedies

Herbal Baths

N.B. Also have a look at the Essential Oils section for further advice on bathing. All the baths suggested for previous age groups are appropriate, but there are some different products that can now be used, and some parents may find them easier and more accessible.

*Rosemary bath for the **morning*** – After a night of illness and fever this bath is really refreshing and restorative. For ease and simplicity, I would recommend using the Weleda Rosemary Bath Milk.

Run a bath as normal for your child, adding two capfuls of Weleda Rosemary Bath Milk. Agitate the water with your hands ensuring that the milk is well distributed in the water. Place your child in the bath.

Alternatively, a rosemary bath using either dried or fresh herbs is just as effective, and perhaps gentler for a sensitive child. To make a herbal bath, please follow the instructions on Herbal Baths in the chapter How to Use the Remedies in this Book.

Use a handful of fresh rosemary, or two tablespoons (or three teabags) of dried rosemary for the herbal brew, and allow the herbs to infuse for 30-40 minutes. Then add the brew to the bath water checking the temperature of the bath before putting the child in.

Allow the child to sit in the herbal bath for 10-15 minutes, or until the child has had enough, but no longer than 20 minutes.

Once the child is out of the bath, dress in fresh clothes and return to rest in bed ensuring they are warm and cosy. Otherwise the child can have a day bed made up on a sofa, and they can be tucked up there to rest after the bath. Make sure the child is kept warm. They will need to rest for at least half an hour.

If your child is not well enough for a bath, or simply doesn't want a bath, a capful of Weleda Bath Milk, or half of the herbal brew can be added to a basin or bowl of warm water, and the child can be washed with a flannel. Alternatively, your child can be washed in bed using an old-fashioned bed-bath technique (for those unfamiliar with the process I explain it in the chapter entitled Practical Nursing Therapies at Home).

Thyme and Chamomile bath in the **evening** – Using either three chamomile teabags and three thyme teabags, or a handful of loose dried chamomile flowers and two tablespoons of dried thyme, or a handful of fresh chamomile flowers and a handful of fresh thyme. Follow the instructions on Herbal Baths in the chapter How to Use the Remedies in this Book.

Allow the herbal brew to infuse for 30-40 minutes and then add it to the bath water (through a sieve to strain out loose herbs if they have been used). Check the temperature of the bath water and follow the same bathing routine as explained for the Rosemary bath above.

Or, using either three chamomile teabags or a handful of chamomile loose tea, follow the instructions on Herbal Baths in the chapter How to Use the Remedies in this Book. Allow the chamomile to infuse in the herbal brew for about 30-45 minutes. Once the bath has been run, add the chamomile herbal brew to the bath (straining if necessary), and then add Weleda Baby and Child Calendula Bath (which has its main ingredient as thyme) to the bath according to manufacturer's instructions. Agitate the water until both the chamomile tea and thyme are well distributed and mixed.

Allow the child to sit in the herbal bath for 10-15 minutes, or until they have had enough. Gently bathe the child in the herbal bath using a flannel or your cupped hands. Try to avoid wetting the child's hair if they have a temperature, as wet hair may chill them once they are out of the bath, and if they have a high temperature having water poured on the head can actually feel quite painful.

Remove the child from the bath and gently pat dry with a towel. Put the child into fresh nightclothes ready for bed. Use *Lemon Legs* or *Lemon Socks* therapy (described later in this chapter) if your baby still needs some help to settle for the night.

12 Months to 3 Years of Age

Herbal Tea

At this age, tea can now be sweetened with honey. Honey has many excellent, health-enhancing properties, especially when the honey is raw and locally sourced. Please see the Glossary of Remedy Ingredients for the medicinal benefits of honey.

Please follow the instructions on Making a Herbal Tea in the chapter How to Use the Remedies in this Book. These are very mild-tasting herbal teas, and traditionally very safe and easy to persuade children to take, even if they are unsweetened.

Lime Flower (also known as Linden Flower) tea – Allow the flowers to infuse for 15 minutes and then remove the herbs or tea bag.

Try to give four to eight teaspoons of the herbal tea (20-40mls) every three hours for up to four doses, (80-160mls) per 12 hour period.

Chamomile tea – This can either be given on its own or combined with the lime flower tea. Allow the chamomile (or chamomile and lime flower combination), to brew for 15 minutes and then remove from the boiled water.

Give four to eight teaspoons of the herbal tea (20-40mls) every three hours for up to four doses, (80-160mls) per 12 hour period.

Elderflower tea – This tea can be used alone or combined for an especially wonderful tonic with both lime flower and chamomile. To brew as a single (or combination) flower infusion, allow the herb/s to infuse for 10-15 minutes in freshly boiled water.

If you don't want to combine the herbs together then you can always alternate the herbs throughout the day. The tea can be sipped day and night.

Herbal Tinctures and Glycerites

I would suggest using the tincture of elderflower and lime flower for fevers, administered by diluting drops in either milk, juice or water with a dosage according to manufacturer's instructions.

A word about Echinacea…

Please see the Glossary of Ingredients for Remedies chapter of this book for more information on echinacea, as in Britain we are theoretically restricted from using or advising use in children under the age of twelve years old.

However, a qualified medical herbalist or herbal apothecary such as Botanica Medica can make an Echinacea glycerite or tincture for your child specifically if you speak to them. You can also make your own tinctures and glycerites at home. Recipes and instructions on how to do this can be found in many of the books suggested in the Resources section.

If you have access to the internet and are happy to order from there, then there are two products I have used with my own children. The first is called Echinature, made by a New Zealand company called Kiwiherb. Their therapeutic formula is suitable to use from the ages of 0-12 years old. It is alcohol free, great-tasting and uses no artificial nasties or added sugars.

Another glycerite of Echinacea, which is easy to order through the internet, is called ChildLife Echinacea. ChildLife is made by a reputable American company and is very easy to administer, tasting slightly of orange. Again, this product also has very pure ingredients and is recommended for use in children from six months of age.

However, as always, I advise using your own judgment and intuition on this matter, and ensure you are well informed. Other mothers, books and qualified herbalists can help guide you towards a decision you feel comfortable with. Always ensure your decisions relating to health come from a place of knowledge rather than fear.

Herbal Syrup

Elderberry (Sambucus Nigra) syrup – This panacea can be bought ready made from health food shops, but it's easy to make yourself. All you will need to make this simple and delicious syrup are elderberries, water and sugar, or now your child is over one year old you can substitute sugar with honey if you wish. The recipe can be found in the chapter on Remedy Recipes.

However, if you do decide to buy elderberry syrup, be aware that many commercial syrups contain preservatives and additional ingredients which may not be beneficial. Ask in your local health food shop for advice, or consult your healthcare practitioner.

12 Months to 3 Years of Age

There are a couple of brands I would recommend at the time of writing this book. Biona do a wonderful Elderberry Juice with nothing added and it is reasonably priced. Children can enjoy it diluted in warm water with honey or maple syrup to sweeten it. It almost has the taste of hot Ribena, which I remember from childhood as a cure-all. Pukka Herbs also do a great elderberry syrup combined with potent herbs and Manuka Honey. It is expensive but it does contain quality ingredients. Pukka elderberry syrup does taste quite strong for children and is often in need of dilution. We use this one in our house for extremely stubborn coughs and colds and dilute it with a little water in a shot glass. Another delicious-tasting, simple elderberry syrup is made in Oxfordshire from locally sourced elderberries and can be ordered online from http://www.dolrosacanina.co.uk.

Dosage for Homemade Elderberry Syrup

Half a teaspoon to one teaspoon (2.5-5mls) mixed with a small amount of water, or added to formula, yoghurt, porridge, fruit purees etc., to be taken up to three times per day during acute illness and fever, usually for a maximum of five days. As a maintenance dose through the winter months half to one teaspoon once per day is usually sufficient.

Essential Oils

Essential Oil Bath

N.B. These can also be used as a flannel wash or bed bath (see Practical Nursing Therapies at Home for instructions), in a sink or bowl. Just halve the quantity of essential oil that is used for a bath.

Rosemary and Bergamot bath for the **morning** – Run a bath as usual for your child. Before placing the child in the bath add two drops of rosemary essential oil and two drops of bergamot essential oil. Agitate the water to ensure oil is well distributed in the bath. Close windows and doors so that the child can benefit from the vapours rising from the steam of the bath, as well as the medicinal properties being absorbed by the skin.

Thyme Linalol and Bergamot bath for the **evening** – Run a bath as usual for your child. Before placing your child in the bath add two drops of Thyme Linalol essential oil and two drops of bergamot essential oil to the bath. Agitate the water to ensure that the oils are well-distributed in the bath water. Close windows and doors so that your child can benefit from the inhaled vapours from the steam of the bath as well as absorbing the therapeutic benefits of the oils through the skin.

N.B. It is very important that it is Thyme Linalol, (Sweet Thyme) that is used and NOT any other type of Thyme such as Thyme Vulgaris. Thyme Linalol is the gentlest essential oil for children and other types of thyme can irritate the skin. The only Thyme Linalol I use is one made by Neal's Yard. If your child has sensitive skin, then please use with caution for the first time.

Lemon oil massage (See chapter on Practical Nursing Therapies at Home for instructions)

Dosage

Two drops of Lemon Essential Oil diluted in a tablespoon of carrier oil (almond or olive oil, etc).

Or, one pump of Dr Hauschka Lemon, Lemongrass Vitalising Oil per leg, or diluted according to the tolerance of the child in a carrier oil such as almond oil, olive oil, etc.

My personal experience is that this remedy is especially useful before bed in the evening. My daughter adores the lemon oil massage, and it helps her to have a restful and comfortable night when she has a fever.

Other Remedies and Treatments

Lemon Socks (See chapter on Practical Nursing Therapies at Home for instructions)

This treatment has been mentioned in the previous age group, along with Lemon Legs, which is suggested for newborns up to six months. You can still use Lemon Legs if you wish, and you can refer back to the previous age group and Practical Nursing Therapies at Home section for instructions.

12 Months to 3 Years of Age

Fever in Age 3 to 5 years old

N.B. Please consult the chapter on Assessing Your Child and the Traffic Light System for fevers in conjunction with this chapter.

If you are ever concerned about a fever in your child, I would always advise consulting a medical professional. Once your child has been seen and a diagnosis given, you can proceed how you wish in terms of supporting your child through illness.

Signs and Symptoms Your Child May Have a Fever

- Feels hot to touch
- Has a faster breathing rate
- Has flushed cheeks
- Has an increased heart rate
- Is more febrile, i.e. grisly, grumpy, crying easily and difficult to comfort
- Is sleepy, complains of being tired, falls asleep at unusual times of day
- Is eating more frequently or less frequently, requesting specific foods
- Rejects food offered
- Is nauseous and/or vomiting
- Complains of feeling cold or hot
- Is clingy
- Complains of headache or stomach ache
- The child has a raised temperature according to the thermometer. A tympanic (ear) thermometer can be used from this age.

Practical Tips

At this age children should be able to communicate whether they are hot or cold, comfortable or not. You will also need to use your observational skills and common sense regarding how to dress your child with a fever, taking into account the ambient heat in the room and if your child appears too hot or is shivering because their body is trying to generate heat to create a fever.

Staying hydrated is vital; however, at this age children are at less risk of dehydration compared to babies. Their bodies are bigger and therefore contain more fluid. Encourage small sips of water or diluted fruit juices and sweetened herbal teas to ensure the child remains well hydrated. This will also provide gentle medicine as well as vital vitamins and minerals to support your child's recovery.

Creating a calm, quiet and peaceful environment that supports and encourages a child to rest is ideal. At this age a child with a fever will often sleep during the day, or fall asleep whilst being read to. Sleep allows the body to heal and undertake the processes vital to regaining health. Don't be tempted to feel that your child needs to be occupied or engaged.

Give plenty of cuddles to the child with Mummy and/or Daddy, and lots of reassurance. Sometimes children this age can feel quite anxious about being ill, especially if the main carer also has anxieties surrounding illness. If you are exhausted from looking after an unwell child, then try to rest when the child rests, and leave non-essential chores until this illness passes and energy levels return.

Homoeopathic Remedies
(See Administering Homeopathic Medicines)

Aconite 6C or 30C The first remedy to go to for sudden onset of symptoms and in the early stages of a fever. The child may feel cold and suffer chills as their body tries to create a fever. The child may not want to be uncovered or undressed because they will feel the cold acutely and shiver. The child will be thirsty and restless.

Belladonna 6C or 30C A common remedy usually given once a fever is established. The characteristics are for unusual restlessness and agitation, particularly at night, and a red, flushed face. Heat is also a distinguishing factor; the head especially feels very hot to touch, with heat almost radiating off the body. In contrast hands and feet can feel cool. Delirium with fever at night is also a feature that would suggest this remedy.

Arsenicum 6C or 30C A child needing Arsenicum will feel chilly and better for being kept warm. They will be restless, anxious and thirsty for small, frequent drinks. Symptoms are usually at their worst between midnight and 2-3am.

3–5 Years of Age

Bryonia 6C or 30C A child needing this remedy would have the heat of fever but with an accompanying dryness of the skin and mucous membranes. A dry mouth and lips are accompanied by a thirst where the child gulps down fluid greedily. Even tiny movements cause the child to cry out in distress.

Pulsatilla 6C or 30C A child needing Pulsatilla will be weepy and need to be soothed by company or being carried and rocked continually. They will want to sleep with the parent and be quite clingy and whiny. A Pulsatilla child will not be thirsty at all and feel much better in the open air, or with access to fresh air. It is especially important that a child needing Pulsatilla is prevented from getting a chill when exposed to fresh air.

Chamomilla 6C or 30C The child is irritable and restless, almost appearing angry or in pain. They may be screaming and crying, feeling hot even on their extremities. They may have hot feet especially, which they don't want covered and will kick covers off. They can't abide heat, or being cold or fresh air; nothing is right and the child is inconsolable unless being carried or rocked. The parent or carer will often feel at a total loss and as if they can't do a thing right for the child.

Nux Vomica 6C or 30C A child needing Nux Vomica has frequently developed a fever as a result of a change in diet, eating rich foods, or lack of sleep. In a young baby, it can be a change from breast milk to formula, or being around a lot of family and being passed from one relative to another. For an older child, it is the classic remedy to give for a fever after a birthday party with lots of excitement, sugary food and drinks. Frequently digestive issues such as diarrhoea or constipation and headaches accompany a fever. The child will feel chilly and want to be covered at all times.

Ferrum Phos. Bio Chemic Tissue Salt This is a good remedy for the early stages of a fever and is the classic remedy for inflammation and slow onset of fever. This is the remedy for fevers with few obvious causes or symptoms. Ferrum Phos is often indicated for fevers that occur after a period of over-exertion, or when a child seems off colour, not quite themselves but with no obvious cause. It is often a useful remedy in recuperation where the child feels tired easily and is generally low in energy.

Combination Homeopathic Remedies

ABC Remedy – This is a simple combination remedy comprising Aconite, Belladonna and Chamomilla, either in 30C or 6C potency. Most homeopathic pharmacies make a version of this. It is available from both Weleda and Helios and can be ordered on their websites. Good local health food shops and pharmacies such as Boots may also stock this remedy. If you can't get hold of it you can dissolve one homeopathic pillule each of Aconite, Belladonna and Chamomilla into some water and give small sips to your child, either from a bottle, with a medicinal dropper or syringe, or a small cup.

This is a great remedy for children with non-specific symptoms and in the early stages of fever. It is extremely effective for teething-related symptoms too when the child is grisly, clingy, fussy and has red cheeks and sore gums and a mild fever. It is a wonderful go-to, catch-all remedy for the busy or confused parent and amateur homeopath alike and is often the first remedy given in our household.

Herbal Remedies

Herbal Baths

N.B. See also Essential Oil section for further advice on bathing. All the baths suggested for previous age groups are appropriate, so please feel free to stay with what works for your child and your family.

Rosemary bath for the **morning** – After a night of illness and fever this bath is really refreshing and restorative. For ease and simplicity, I would recommend using the Weleda Rosemary Bath Milk.

Run a bath as normal for your child, adding two capfuls of the Weleda Rosemary Bath Milk. Agitate the water with your hands ensuring that the milk is well distributed in the water. Place your child in the bath.

Alternatively, a rosemary bath using either dried or fresh herbs is just as effective, and perhaps gentler for a sensitive child. To make a herbal bath please follow the instructions on Herbal Baths in the chapter How to Use the Remedies in this Book.

Use a handful of fresh rosemary, or two tablespoons (or three teabags) of dried rosemary for the herbal brew, and allow the herbs to infuse for 30-40 minutes. Then add the brew to the bath water checking the temperature of the bath before putting the child in.

Allow the child to sit in the herbal bath for 10-15 minutes, or until the child has had enough, but no longer than 20 minutes.

Once the child is out of the bath, dress them in fresh clothes and return them to bed ensuring they are warm and cosy. Otherwise the child can have a day bed made up on a sofa, and they can be tucked up there to rest after the bath. Make sure the child is kept warm. They will need to rest for at least half an hour.

If your child is not well enough for a bath, or simply doesn't want a bath, a capful of Weleda bath milk, or half of the herbal brew can be added to a basin or bowl of warm water, and the child can be washed with a flannel. Alternatively, your child can be washed in bed using an old-fashioned bed bath technique (for those unfamiliar with the process I explain it in the chapter entitled Practical Nursing Therapies at Home).

Thyme and Chamomile bath in the **evening** – Using either three chamomile teabags and three thyme teabags, or a handful of loose dried chamomile flowers and two tablespoons of dried thyme, or a handful of fresh chamomile flowers and a handful of fresh thyme, follow the instructions on Herbal Baths in the chapter How to Use the Remedies in this Book.

Allow the herbal brew to infuse for 30-40 minutes and then add it to the bath water (through a sieve to strain out loose herbs if they have been used).

Or, using either three chamomile teabags or a handful of chamomile loose tea, follow the instructions on Herbal Baths in the chapter How to Use the Remedies in this Book. Allow the chamomile to infuse in the herbal brew for about 30-45 minutes. Once the bath has been run, add the chamomile herbal brew to the bath (straining if necessary), and then add Weleda Baby and Child Calendula Bath (which has its main ingredient as thyme) to the bath according to manufacturer's instructions. Agitate the water until both the chamomile tea and thyme are well distributed and mixed.

Allow the child to sit in the herbal bath for 10-15 minutes, or until they have had enough. Gently bathe the child in the herbal bath using a flannel or your cupped hands. Try to avoid wetting the child's hair if they have a temperature, as wet hair may chill them once they are out of the bath, and if they have a high temperature having water poured on the head can actually feel quite painful.

Remove the child from the bath and gently pat dry with a towel. Put the child into fresh nightclothes ready for bed. Use *Lemon Legs* or *Lemon Socks* therapy (described later in this chapter) if your child still needs some help to settle for the night.

Herbal Tea

At this age, tea can now be sweetened with honey or maple syrup. Honey has many excellent, health-enhancing properties, especially when the honey is raw and locally sourced. Please see the Glossary of Remedy Ingredients for the medicinal benefits of honey and maple syrup.

Please follow the instructions on Making a Herbal Tea in the chapter How to Use the Remedies in this Book. These are very mild-tasting herbal teas, and traditionally very safe and easy to persuade children to take, even if they are unsweetened.

Lime Flower (also known as Linden Flower) tea – Allow the flowers to infuse for 15 minutes and then remove the herbs or tea bag.

Try to give 60-100mls of the herbal tea (two to three espresso sized cups approximately) every three hours for up to four doses per 12 hour period.

Chamomile tea – This can either be given on its own or combined with the lime flower Tea. If you decide to combine the two teas, simply add a teaspoon or teabag of chamomile flowers to the teaspoon or teabag of lime flowers. Allow the herbs to brew for 15 minutes.

Try to give 60-100mls of the herbal tea (two to three espresso sized cups approximately) every three hours for up to four doses per 12 hour period.

Elderflower tea – This tea can be used alone or combined for an especially wonderful tonic with both lime flower and chamomile. To brew as a single (or combination) flower infusion, allow the herb/s to infuse for 10-15 minutes in freshly boiled water.

If you don't want to combine the herbs together then you can always alternate the herbs throughout the day. The tea can be sipped day and night.

Herbal Tinctures and Glycerites

Tincture of Elderflower and/or Lime Flower – To be administered according to manufacturer's instructions.

Please see the Resources section of the book for suggested outlets that make excellent quality tinctures. Alternatively, you can make your own, and there are plenty of wonderful wise women who have published books with recipes and step-by-step instructions on how to do this. Again, I refer you to the Resources section where I have listed my favourites, although there are many others.

Glycerite or tincture of Echinacea – Please see the Glossary of Ingredients for Remedies chapter of this book for more information on echinacea; in Britain we are theoretically restricted from using or advising generic use in children under the age of twelve years old. However, if you feel comfortable administering echinacea either as a glycerite or tincture to your child I would advise consulting a qualified medical herbalist or herbal pharmacy to obtain a correct dosage for your child and a well-made medicine.

Botanica Medica in the U.K. make a wonderful *Immune Glycerite*, suitable for this age range that tastes delicious and contains both echinacea and elderberry – perfect! Botanica Medica are a reputable herbal apothecary who offer free consultations over the phone and send medicine in the post that arrives the next day. Please see the Resources section for contact details. The singular drawback is that the products are on the expensive side, but the quality is unsurpassed.

Otherwise you are always free to make a tincture, tea or glycerite yourself and I have included books with recipes in the Resources section.

Via the magic of the internet, or friends and relatives overseas, you may be able to obtain the following reputable products – and if you are fortunate enough to live in a country where they are sold, take a stroll to your local Health Food shop—you lucky people!

Echinature – Suitable for newborns to 12 year olds. Manufactured in New Zealand by the brilliant Kiwiherb.

ChildLife Echinacea – Suitable from 6 months of age until 12 years old. Manufactured for ChildLife in Los Angeles, U.S.A.

3–5 Years of Age

Herbal Syrup

Elderberry (Sambucus Nigra) syrup – This panacea can be bought ready-made from Health Food shops or online, but it's easy to make yourself. However, if you do decide to buy elderberry syrup, be aware that many commercial syrups contain added ingredients and preservatives. Always check the ingredients list. Ask in your local health food shop for advice, or consult your healthcare practitioner.

There are some well-known brands making wonderful elderberry syrups, some containing added herbs for additional health benefits. I would suggest keeping the flavours simple with children and perhaps trying a few to find a family favourite. We enjoy Biona elderberry juice, Pukka elderberry syrup (perhaps a bit strong-tasting for some kids!) and a delicious, simple syrup made with reduced sugar from a farm in Oxfordshire, available online from http://www.dolrosacanina.co.uk.

If you do decide to make your own elderberry syrup, all you will need are elderberries, water and sugar, or as your child is over one year old you can substitute sugar with honey if you wish. The recipe can be found in the chapter on Remedy Recipes.

Dosage for Homemade Elderberry Syrup

One teaspoon (5mls) mixed with a small amount of water, or added to yoghurt, porridge etc. and to be taken up to three times per day during acute illness and fever, usually for 5-10 days. As a maintenance dose through the winter months, one teaspoon once per day is usually sufficient.

Lime Flower syrup – This has the same medicinal properties as lime flower tea, but may be more palatable in this form for a child. It has a lot of sugar though, especially if combined with other syrups. I have only seen this syrup available online from http://www.dolrosacanina.co.uk.

The only reason I have suggested this syrup here is that the sugar content may not be ideal for a younger child. This is, of course, a matter for parental discretion. Dosage is according to the manufacturer's instructions, or dilute the syrup as you would a cordial and encourage your child to sip regularly.

Essential Oils

Essential Oil Bath

N.B. These can also be used as a flannel wash or bed bath in a sink or bowl. Just halve the quantity of essential oil that is used for a bath.

Rosemary and Bergamot bath for the **morning** – Run a bath as usual for your child. Before placing the child in the bath add three drops of rosemary essential oil and three drops of bergamot essential oil. Agitate the water to ensure oil is well distributed in the bath. Close windows and doors so that the child can benefit from the vapours rising from the steam of the bath, as well as some medicinal properties being absorbed by the skin.

Thyme Linalol and Bergamot bath for the **evening** – Run a bath as usual for your child. Before placing your child in the bath add three drops of Thyme Linalol essential oil and three drops of bergamot essential oil to the bath. Agitate the water to ensure that the oils are well-distributed in the bath water. Close windows and doors so that your child can benefit from the inhaled vapours from the steam of the bath as well as absorbing the therapeutic benefits of the oils through the skin.

N.B. It is very important that it is Thyme Linalol, (Sweet Thyme) that is used and NOT any other type of Thyme such as Thyme Vulgaris. Thyme Linalol is the gentlest essential oil for children and other types of Thyme can irritate the skin. The only Thyme Linalol I use is one made by Neal's Yard. If your child has sensitive skin, then please use with caution for the first time.

Rosemary spritzer – Use a glass bottle with a spray head. You may have one at home or they can be ordered off any aromatherapy website. If you are using a bottle from home, make sure it is clean and that any previous contents of the bottle aren't toxic or dangerous. Fill the bottle with 50mls of water and add three drops of rosemary essential oil to the bottle. Shake well before each use and spray liberally on the arms and legs and feet (avoiding the face) of your child throughout the day if they are feeling or appear uncomfortably hot with fever. It should deliver a cooling mist to your child with a fresh aroma. A drop or two of lemon essential oil can also be added to the mixture.

3–5 Years of Age

Rosemary and Lavender compress – A compress is a very simple way to soothe, cool and refresh a child with a fever.

Soak two flannels in lukewarm/body temperature water, then squeeze excess water out so that the flannel doesn't drip. Fold one flannel to fit on the forehead of the child and one to fit on the back of the neck of the child. Place one drop of rosemary and one drop of lavender essential oil on one side of each of the two flannels and place the essential oil side of the flannel against the skin; one flannel on the forehead, the other flannel on the back of the neck. The oils will penetrate the skin imparting their medicinal benefits, the aroma will refresh the spirit, and the coolness of the flannel will soothe the child and increase their sense of comfort.

Lemon Oil massage (See chapter on Practical Nursing Therapies at Home for instructions)

My personal experience is that this remedy is especially useful after an evening bath and before bed. It calms and soothes, enabling rest whilst allowing a fever to serve its purpose.

Lemon socks can be added later in the night if the child becomes hot and restless, but this treatment usually works for the first half of the night on its own, and frequently until morning.

Dosage

Two drops of Lemon Essential Oil diluted in a tablespoon of carrier oil (almond or olive oil, etc).

Or, one pump of Dr Hauschka Lemon, Lemongrass Vitalising Oil per leg, or diluted according to the tolerance of the child in a carrier oil such as almond oil, olive oil, etc.

Other Remedies and Treatments

Lemon Socks
(See chapter on *Practical Nursing Therapies At Home for instructions*)

This treatment helps to lower a fever just enough to help keep a child comfortable through the night, without impacting on the vital role fever plays in fighting infection. Lemon Socks has been mentioned in the previous age group,

3–5 Years of Age

along with Lemon Legs, which is suggested for newborns up to six months. You can still use Lemon Legs if you wish, and you can refer back to the previous age group and Practical Nursing Therapies at Home section for instructions.

3–5 Years of Age

Fever in Age 5 to 12 years old

N.B. Please consult the chapter on Assessing Your Child and the Traffic Light System for fevers in conjunction with this chapter.

At this stage your child should be able to recognise if they are feeling unwell, and should be able to communicate quite clearly what their symptoms are. If you are ever concerned about a fever in your child, I would always advise consulting a medical professional. Once your child has been seen and a diagnosis given you can proceed how you wish in terms of supporting your child through illness.

You may find that some of this section repeats what the previous sections for younger ages have suggested, however the dosages are different. There are some subtle changes and tweaks, building on the foundation of knowledge and remedies we have explored in previous chapters.

Signs and Symptoms Your Child May Have a Fever

- Feels hot to touch
- Has a faster breathing rate
- Has flushed cheeks or a pale pallor
- Has an increased heart rate
- Is more febrile, i.e. grisly, grumpy, crying easily
- Is fatigued, complains of being tired, falls asleep at unusual times of day
- Is eating less frequently, requesting specific foods
- Rejects food offered
- Is nauseous and/or vomiting
- Complains of feeling cold or hot
- Is clingy
- Complains of headache or stomach ache
- The child has a raised temperature according to the thermometer. A tympanic (ear) thermometer can be used. I would advise taking the temperature in both ears to begin with until your confidence builds.

Practical Tips

The older children get the more efficiently their bodies should cope with fever, especially if they have been allowed to experience fever without pharmaceutical intervention. When they are over five years of age, you should notice a reduced need to offer interventions to enhance comfort. Rest and hydration should be the main focus of care, and treat a fever with remedies in this book only as and when required. A bath in the morning and evening with some essential oils and a soothing, restful and healing environment are really the mainstay of care as children grow up.

At this age, children should be able to communicate if they are feeling hot or cold, and should be able to add/remove clothing and bedding as needed. With younger children, it is still advisable to monitor clothing and bedding to make sure they don't get chilled or over heat.

I continue to advocate frequent, small sips of water, diluted fruit juices or herbal teas that will help provide gentle medicine as well as vitamins and minerals to support your child's recovery. Ensure your child remains well-hydrated, but dehydration from fever is less of a concern at this age than with a baby. If your child is showing signs of an appetite for food, then making simple, easily digested meals such as soup and jelly is a good idea. Please see Recipes During Illness for some suggestions.

If the child is not ill enough to stay in bed, then quiet activities such as using modelling clay or play dough, building with Lego or painting or colouring and being read to, are all therapeutic activities. My children tend to regress a bit when they are unwell, so they want to do things which they would have done a lot when they were younger, like their baby jigsaws, or play with their old Brio train set. Older children may enjoy a magazine, audiobooks, podcasts or just sleeping.

Give plenty of cuddles to the child, and lots of reassurance. Older children especially need affection when they are ill, as they may be at an age when they are starting to push parents away and reach for independence when they are well. When illness strikes, personal barriers are down and we are at our most vulnerable, use this time to rebuild closeness, affection and trust with older children.

Homoeopathic Remedies
(See *Administering Homeopathic Medicines*)

Aconite 6C or 30C The first remedy to go to for sudden onset of symptoms and in the early stages of a fever. The child may feel cold and suffer chills as their body tries to create a fever. The child may not want to be uncovered or undressed because they will feel the cold acutely and shiver. The child will be thirsty and restless.

Belladonna 6C or 30C A common remedy usually given once a fever is established. The characteristics are for unusual restlessness and agitation, particularly at night, and a red, flushed face. Heat is also a distinguishing factor; the head especially feels very hot to touch, with heat almost radiating off the body. In contrast hands and feet can feel cool. Delirium with fever at night is also a feature that would suggest this remedy.

Arsenicum 6C or 30C A child needing Arsenicum will feel chilly and better for being kept warm. They will be restless, anxious and thirsty for small, frequent drinks. Symptoms are usually at their worst between midnight and 2-3am.

Bryonia 6C or 30C A child needing this remedy would have the heat of fever but with an accompanying dryness of the skin and mucous membranes. A dry mouth and lips are accompanied by a thirst where the child gulps down fluid greedily. Even tiny movements cause the child to cry out in distress.

Pulsatilla 6C or 30C A child needing Pulsatilla will be weepy and need to be soothed by company. They may want to sleep with the parent and be quite clingy and whiny. A Pulsatilla child will not be thirsty at all and feel much better in the open air, or with access to fresh air. It is especially important that a child needing Pulsatilla is prevented from getting a chill when exposed to fresh air.

Chamomilla 6C or 30C The child is irritable and restless, almost appearing angry or in pain. They may be screaming and crying, feeling hot even on their extremities. They may have hot feet especially, which they don't want covered and will kick covers off. They can't abide heat, or being cold or fresh air; nothing is right and the child is inconsolable. The parent or carer will often feel at a total loss and as if they can't do a thing right for the child.

Nux Vomica 6C or 30C A child needing Nux Vomica has frequently developed a fever as a result of a change in diet, eating rich foods, or lack of sleep. For an older child, it is the classic remedy to give for a fever after a birthday party with lots of excitement, sugary food and drinks. Frequently digestive issues such as diarrhoea or constipation and headaches accompany a fever. The child will feel chilly and want to be covered at all times.

Ferrum Phos. Bio Chemic Tissue Salt This is a good remedy for the early stages of a fever and is the classic remedy for inflammation and slow onset of fever. This is the remedy for fevers with few obvious causes or symptoms. Ferrum Phos is often indicated for fevers that occur after a period of over-exertion, or when a child seems off colour, not quite themselves but with no obvious cause. It is often a useful remedy in recuperation where the child feels tired easily and is generally low in energy.

Combination Homeopathic Remedies

ABC Remedy – This is a simple combination remedy comprising Aconite, Belladonna and Chamomilla, either in 30C or 6C potency. Most homeopathic pharmacies make a version of this. It is available from both Weleda and Helios and can be ordered on their websites. Good local health food shops and pharmacies such as Boots may also stock this remedy. If you can't get hold of it, you can dissolve one homeopathic pillule each of Aconite, Belladonna and Chamomilla into some water and give small sips to your child, either from a bottle, with a medicinal dropper or syringe, or a small cup.

This is a great remedy for children with non-specific symptoms and in the early stages of fever. It is extremely effective for teething-related symptoms too when the child is grisly, clingy, fussy and has red cheeks and sore gums and a mild fever. It is a wonderful go-to, catch-all remedy for the busy or confused parent and amateur homeopath alike and is often the first remedy given in our household.

Herbal Remedies

Herbal Baths

N.B. See also Essential Oil section for further advice on bathing

All the baths suggested for previous age groups are appropriate, so please feel free to stay with what works for your child and your family.

To make a herbal bath please follow the instructions on Herbal Baths in the chapter How to Use the Remedies in this Book.

Rosemary bath for the **morning** – After a night of illness and fever this bath is really refreshing and restorative. For ease and simplicity, I would recommend using Weleda Rosemary Bath Milk.

Run a bath as normal for your child, adding two capfuls of Weleda Rosemary Bath Milk. Agitate the water with your hands ensuring that the milk is well distributed in the water. Place your child in the bath.

Alternatively, a rosemary bath using either dried or fresh herbs is just as effective, and perhaps gentler for a sensitive child. To make a herbal bath please follow the instructions on Herbal Baths in the chapter How to Use the Remedies in this Book.

Use a handful of fresh rosemary, or two tablespoons (or three teabags) of dried rosemary for the herbal brew, and allow the herbs to infuse for 30-40 minutes. Then add the brew to the bath water, checking the temperature of the bath before putting the child in.

Allow the child to sit in the herbal bath for 10-15 minutes, or until the child has had enough, but no longer than 20 minutes.

Once the child is out of the bath, dress in fresh clothes and return to bed ensuring they are warm and cosy to rest. Otherwise the child can have a day bed made up on a sofa, and they can be tucked up there to rest after the bath. Make sure the child is kept warm. They will need to rest for at least half an hour.

If your child is not well enough for a bath, or simply doesn't want a bath, a capful of Weleda bath milk, or half of the herbal brew can be added to a basin or bowl of warm water, and the child can be washed with a flannel. Alternatively, your child can be washed in bed using an old-fashioned bed-bath technique (for those unfamiliar with the process I explain it in the chapter entitled Practical Nursing Therapies at Home).

5–12 Years of Age

*Thyme and Chamomile bath in the **evening*** – Using either three chamomile teabags and three thyme teabags, or a handful of loose dried chamomile flowers and two tablespoons of dried thyme, or a handful of fresh chamomile flowers and a handful of fresh thyme, follow the instructions on Herbal Baths in the chapter How to Use the Remedies in this Book.

Allow the herbal brew to infuse for 30-40 minutes and then add it to the bath water (through a sieve to strain out loose herbs if they have been used).

Or, using either three chamomile teabags or a handful of chamomile loose tea, follow the instructions on Herbal Baths in the chapter How to Use the Remedies in this Book. Allow the chamomile to infuse in the herbal brew for about 30-45 minutes. Once the bath has been run, add the chamomile herbal brew to the bath (straining if necessary), and then add Weleda Baby and Child Calendula Bath (which has thyme as its main ingredient) to the bath according to manufacturer's instructions. Agitate the water until both the chamomile tea and thyme are well distributed and mixed.

Allow the child to sit in the herbal bath for 10-15 minutes, or until they have had enough. Gently bathe the child in the herbal bath using a flannel or your cupped hands. Try to avoid wetting the child's hair if they have a temperature, as wet hair may chill them once they are out of the bath, and if they have a high temperature having water poured on the head can actually feel quite painful.

Remove the child from the bath and gently pat dry with a towel. Put the child into fresh nightclothes ready for bed. Use *Lemon Legs* or *Lemon Socks* therapy (described later in this chapter) if your child still needs some help to settle for the night.

Herbal Tea

At this age, tea can be sweetened with honey or maple syrup. Honey has many excellent, health enhancing properties, and it is worth spending a little more on good quality honey, and avoiding generic super market honey. Honey sold in supermarkets has often been heat-treated and processed, and sometimes diluted with sugar to reduce the costs. See the Glossary of Ingredients for Remedies for more information about honey and maple syrup.

Lime Flower (also known as linden flower) tea – Allow the flowers to infuse for 15 minutes and then remove the herbs or tea bag.

From the age of five until eight years old (inclusive) try to give a half a normal sized mug (125mls) of herbal tea every three hours, or over a three hour period for up to four times a day.

From the age of nine and upwards, try to encourage the child to drink a whole mug (250mls) of herbal tea every three hours for up to four times per day.

Elderflower tea – This tea can be used alone or combined for an especially wonderful tonic with both lime flower and chamomile. To brew as a single, (or combination) flower infusion, allow the herb/s to infuse for 10-15 minutes in freshly boiled water.

If you don't want to combine the herbs together then you can always alternate the herbs throughout the day. The tea can be sipped day and night.

From the age of five until eight years old (inclusive) try to give a half a normal sized mug (125mls) of herbal tea every three hours, or over a three hour period for up to four times a day.

From the age of nine and upwards, try to encourage the child to drink a whole mug (250mls) of herbal tea every three hours for up to four times per day.

Drinking this amount of tea can be encouraged using small, special glasses, special cups or mugs. Also, I suggest making up a jug of iced herbal tea to sip during the day. I have been known to add straws, fruit (like a Pimms), umbrellas and all sorts of cocktail paraphernalia to an iced herbal tea to encourage consumption! See the Recipes During Illness for suggestions.

Herbal Tinctures and Glycerites

Tincture of Elderflower and/or Lime Flower – To be administered according to manufacturer's instructions.

Please see the Resources section of the book for suggested outlets that make and sell excellent quality tinctures. There are also a number of books suggested under Resources that can guide you on how to make your own tinctures, glycerites, teas and remedies should you be so inclined.

A word about Echinacea…

I am writing this book in Britain where it is suggested not to recommend echinacea for use in children under 12 years of age. Please see the chapter on the Glossary of Ingredients for Remedies for further information so you can make an informed choice on the matter.

For those of you who are happy to use echinacea, or who have already done so, there are three products I can recommend having used them with my own children. If you are at all unsure about using echinacea, then I suggest contacting a qualified Medical Herbalist or Herbal Pharmacy and Apothecary where you can obtain sensible, unbiased advice (see Resources section).

Immune Glycerite – Specifically formulated for children in the UK, this glycerite is very delicious. It contains elderberry AND echinacea and is available from Botanica Medica (see Resources for contact details). They can post the medicine to you and will give free advice over the telephone.

The following products are available online, but can be easily bought in America, Australia and New Zealand in local Health Food shops.

Echinature – Suitable for newborns to 12 year olds. Manufactured in New Zealand by the brilliant Kiwiherb.

ChildLife Echinacea – Suitable from six months of age until 12 years old. Manufactured for ChildLife in Los Angeles, U.S.A.

You can also try making your own; have a look at the books I recommend in the Resources section for ideas and recipes, or seek recommendations from friends or herbalists.

Herbal Syrup

Elderberry (Sambucus Nigra) syrup – This panacea can be bought ready-made from Health Food shops or online, but it's easy to make yourself. However, if you do decide to buy elderberry syrup, be aware that many commercial syrups contain added ingredients and preservatives. Always check the ingredients list. Ask in your local health food shop for advice, or consult your healthcare practitioner.

There are some well-known brands making wonderful elderberry syrups, some containing added herbs for additional health benefits. I would suggest keeping the flavours simple with children and perhaps trying a few to find a family favourite. We enjoy Biona elderberry juice, Pukka elderberry syrup (perhaps a bit strong-tasting for some kids!) and a delicious, simple syrup made with reduced sugar from a farm in Oxfordshire, available online from http://www.dolrosacanina.co.uk. There are an infinite number to try out there though, so don't be limited by my suggestions, and let me know of any good ones you find along the way!

If you do decide to make your own elderberry syrup, all you will need are elderberries, water and sugar, or as your child is over one year old you can substitute sugar with honey if you wish. The recipe can be found in the chapter on Remedy Recipes.

Dosage for Homemade Elderberry Syrup
One teaspoon (5ml) mixed with a small amount of water, or added to yoghurt, porridge etc. and to be taken up to three times per day during acute illness and fever, usually for a maximum of five days. As a maintenance dose through the winter months one to two teaspoons (5-10ml) once per day is usually sufficient.

Lime Flower syrup – This has the same medicinal properties as lime flower tea, but may be more palatable in this form for a child. It is a lot of sugar though, especially if combined with other syrups. I have only seen this syrup available online from http://www.dolrosacanina.co.uk.

The only reason I have suggested this syrup here is that the sugar content may not be ideal for a younger child. This is of course a matter for parental discretion. Dosage is according to the manufacturer's instructions, or dilute the syrup as you would a cordial and encourage your child to sip regularly.

Essential Oils

Essential Oil Bath

N.B. These can also be used as a flannel wash or bed bath in a sink or bowl. Just halve the quantity of essential oil that is used for a bath.

Rosemary and Bergamot bath for the **morning** – Run a bath as usual for your child. Before placing the child in the bath add three drops of rosemary essential oil and three drops of bergamot essential oil. Agitate the water to ensure oil is well distributed in the bath. Close windows and doors so that the child can benefit from the vapours rising from the steam of the bath, as well as medicinal benefits being absorbed by the skin.

Thyme Linalol and Bergamot bath for the **evening** – Run a bath as usual for your child. Before placing your child in the bath add three drops of Thyme Linalol essential oil and three drops of bergamot essential oil to the bath. Agitate the water to ensure that the oils are well-distributed in the bath water. Close windows and doors so that your child can benefit from the inhaled vapours from the steam of the bath as well as absorbing the therapeutic benefits of the oils through the skin.

   N.B. It is very important that it is Thyme Linalol, (Sweet Thyme) that is used and NOT any other type of Thyme such as Thyme Vulgaris. Thyme Linalol is the gentlest essential oil for children and other types of Thyme can irritate the skin. The only Thyme Linalol I use is one made by Neal's Yard. If your child has sensitive skin, then please use with caution for the first time.

Rosemary spritzer – Use a glass bottle with a spray head. You may have one at home or they can be ordered off any aromatherapy website. If you are using a bottle from home, make sure it is clean and that any previous contents of the bottle weren't toxic or dangerous. Fill the bottle with 50ml of water and add three drops of rosemary essential oil to the bottle. Shake well before each use and spray liberally on the arms and legs and feet (avoiding the face) of your child throughout the day if they are feeling or appear uncomfortably hot with fever. It should deliver a cooling mist to your child with a fresh aroma. A drop of lemon essential oil can also be added to the mixture.

Rosemary and Lavender compress – A compress is a very simple way to soothe, cool and refresh a child with a fever.

   Soak two flannels in lukewarm/body temperature water, then squeeze excess water out so that the flannel doesn't drip. Fold one flannel to fit on the forehead of the child and one to fit on the back of the neck of the child. Place one drop of rosemary and one drop of lavender essential oil on one side of each of the two flannels and place the essential oil side of the flannel against the skin; one flannel on the forehead, the other flannel on the back of the neck.

5–12 Years of Age

The oils will penetrate the skin imparting their medicinal benefits, the aroma will refresh the spirit, and the coolness of the flannel will soothe the child and increase their sense of comfort.

Lemon Oil massage (See chapter on Practical Nursing Therapies at Home for instructions)

This remedy is especially effective after an evening bath and before bed. It helps to calm and soothe the child, ensuring restorative sleep through the night.

Lemon socks can be added later in the night if the child becomes hot and restless, but the Lemon Oil treatment usually works for the first half of the night on its own, and frequently until morning.

Dosage

Two drops of lemon essential oil diluted in a tablespoon of carrier oil (almond or olive oil etc.).

Or

One pump of Dr Hauschka Lemon, Lemongrass Vitalising Oil per leg, or diluted according to the tolerance of the child in a carrier oil such as almond oil, olive oil, etc.

Other Remedies and Treatments

Lemon Socks
(See chapter on *Practical Nursing Therapies at Home for instructions*)

This treatment helps to lower a fever just enough to help keep a child comfortable through the night, without impacting on the vital role fever plays in fighting infection. Lemon Socks has been mentioned in the previous age group, along with Lemon Legs, which is suggested for newborns up to six months. You can still use Lemon Legs if you wish, and you can refer back to the previous age group and Practical Nursing Therapies at Home section for instructions.

Chapter Seven

Practical Nursing Therapies at Home

Giving a Bed Bath

You will need:

- Fresh clothing for the child to wear after the bed bath
- Two large dry towels
- A dry hand towel
- A flannel
- A bowl of warm water with the chosen herbal remedies or essential oils added

How to give a bed bath:

- Start by gathering everything on the list that you need so that you have everything close to hand, then help your child to undress.
- Place one large dry towel under the child in bed, and cover the child with a further large dry towel, ensuring no limbs are exposed and that the child is totally covered and warm from the neck down.
- Have a dry hand towel next to you, a bowl of warm water with the herbal remedies or essential oils added and a flannel as well as the fresh clothing for the child to get into after being washed.
- First gently wash the child's face and the back of the neck, which can get sweaty with a fever in the night. Dry gently with the clean hand towel.

- Then gently fold the large towel back to expose just one hand and arm. Wash the hand and arm and under the armpit with the flannel. Dry the hand, arm and armpit of the child and re-cover with the large dry towel. Repeat on the other side.
- If your child is able to, ask them to roll onto their side so you can wash their back. Pat their back dry gently with the hand towel and then they can roll back.
- Once the top half of the child is done, you can put on fresh clothing such as a pyjama top, vest, t-shirt or nightdress, but don't pull it down further than the navel or belly button. Cover the child once again with the large towel once this has been done.
- Gently fold back the large towel to expose one leg and foot. Wash the foot and wash up the leg using gentle strokes up the calf and thigh. This helps with circulation. Dry the foot and leg and re-cover the child. Repeat on the other side.
- Now fold the large towel down from the shoulders to the thigh so that the child is covered from the thigh downwards. Their top half should be dressed, and their groin and genitals exposed. Wash this area as you would normally if they are a baby or toddler, otherwise if they are old enough I would encourage them to wash this area themselves, and pat dry gently. Dress the child in nappies or underwear and the rest of their clean clothes. Remove towels from under the child, and those covering the child. Cover the child with bedding ensuring they are warm and allow them to rest.

Lemon Socks

Caution: Do not use this therapy on broken or irritated skin and do not use if your child is showing signs of a rising fever, e.g. shivering or showing signs of feeling cold. This therapy is for use when the child feels hot and a fever has spiked. This therapy is to make the child feel more comfortable by enabling the body to decrease a fever fractionally without impeding the immune response.

Place an absorbent mat in the cot or bed under the child's legs, or a thickly folded towel will do. This stops the sheets and mattress getting wet.

Ideally a pair of cotton socks should be used for this treatment plus a pair of wool socks. However, if no wool socks are to hand, then feel free to either improvise with a further pair of cotton socks, or you may feel that just a single pair of lemon socks suffices. It is entirely up to you, depending on what you have to hand and the tolerance of your child.

In a bowl squeeze the juice of a whole fresh lemon (or lime if no lemons are available), which is approximately two tablespoons of juice. I leave the lemons in the water once they have been squeezed. If neither lemons nor limes are to hand it is possible to substitute with one tablespoon of vinegar, although vinegar has quite a strong smell, and babies and children have been known to object to the odour. Mix in 800mls of warm (just slightly warmer than body temperature) water run straight from the tap. Mix well by stirring.

Soak the pair of cotton socks in the lemon water and remove, carefully wringing out excess liquid. The socks should be damp/wet, but not dripping wet. Apply the socks to the feet. Then cover these wet socks ideally with a pair of dry woollen socks, or a pair of dry cotton socks if woollen ones are not available. This slows the evaporation and heat exchange process, ensuring that it is gentle and that the fever doesn't drop too much or too rapidly. However, if no second pair of socks is available, I understand that many parents and practitioners advocate just using the one pair of lemon socks, and not covering with a second layer. I am following the anthroposophic guidance for this remedy by including the second layer, as to me it seems a more effective and gentle cooling process for the body and my children have preferred it. However, you can use your own intuition and what you have to hand to determine your choices for this treatment.

Once the socks have been applied ensure the mattress cover is in the correct place to prevent the mattress and sheets from getting wet and cover the child with appropriate bedding. Keep the lemon juice mixture to hand as it can be reused to soak socks in throughout the night. A fresh batch of lemon juice and water will need to be made each evening.

Lemon Legs

Caution: Do not use this therapy on broken or irritated skin and do not use if your child is showing signs of a rising fever, e.g. shivering or showing signs of feeling cold. This therapy is for use when the child feels hot and a fever has spiked. This therapy *is to make the child feel more comfortable by enabling the body to decrease a fever fractionally without impeding the immune response.*

Place an absorbent mat in the cot or bed, or a thickly folded towel will do. This stops the sheets and mattress getting wet.

Cut or fold a muslin or use plain cotton wool, or even a soft folded flannel, large enough to form a decent compress over the baby's calf area. The cotton wool or muslin would need to be the approximate thickness of 0.3-0.5cm when wet, a decent pad size.

Once you have got the materials cut or folded to the required size and shape, you will also need an old pair of baby tights with the feet and waist cut off so they resemble leg warmers. Alternatively, the legs of baby leggings can be cut off too, or the arms of jumpers or cardigans that are no longer needed. The point of these is to put them on the baby's legs, covering the muslin or cotton wool to hold the lemon compress in place, so they will need to be snug without being tight and cutting off or restricting the circulation of the baby.

In a bowl squeeze the juice of a whole fresh lemon (or lime), which is approximately two tablespoons of juice. If neither lemons nor limes are to hand it is possible to substitute with one tablespoon of vinegar, although vinegar has quite a strong smell, and babies and children have been known to object to the odour. Mix in 500-800mls of warm, just slightly warmer than body temperature water, which can be run straight from the tap. Mix well by stirring.

Soak the muslin or cotton wool in the mixture and remove, carefully wringing out excess liquid. The compress should be wet but not dripping wet. Apply the compress to the lower legs, paying particular attention to covering the calf area. Put the leggings over the top to hold the compress in place.

Place your baby in the cot or bed ensuring that the mattress and bed are protected from getting wet, and cover the child with appropriate bedding. Keep the lemon juice mixture to hand as it can be reused to re-soak the compresses throughout the night. A fresh batch of lemon juice and water will need to be made each evening.

Lemon Oil Massage

Caution: *Do not use this therapy if your child has broken skin. If your child has very sensitive skin then use half the recommended amount of essential oil or dilute the*

Dr. Hauschka Lemon, Lemongrass Vitalising Body oil in either olive or almond oil until it is tolerable for the child.

Prepare the bedroom first by laying a large towel on the bed, and have a large towel to hand to place over the top of the child, and a cover – either a blanket or duvet, to place over the top of the large towel to cover the child at the end of the treatment. Have your oils to hand, either a carrier oil, for example almond oil or olive oil, and lemon essential oil, or the Dr. Hauschka Lemon, Lemongrass Vitalising Body Oil. Dilute or mix them together as required and have them ready in a small bowl or jug.

Following a bath, preferably a herbal bath recommended earlier in the section, take the child out of the bath and wrap in a large towel without drying. Lie the child down on top of the towel already laid on the bed. Cover the child, who should still be wrapped in the towel from the bath, with the extra towel ready by the bed. Expose one leg from the knee downward, ensuring that the rest of the body is covered. Use a teaspoon (5mls approximately) of your ready diluted oils and warm the oil in the palm of your hands before gently applying oils with a slow, stroking action from the toes up to the knee. Repeat to the soles of the feet, up the back of the calf and back of the knee. Add more oil to the palms of your hands if necessary and continue this slow, gentle stroking massage for about one to two minutes. Cover the leg and move to expose the other lower leg to repeat the same process.

Once the lemon oil has been applied, place socks on the feet and cover the child with a blanket or duvet. Allow the child to rest for half an hour before removing the blanket and towels and dressing in night clothes and preparing the child for bed.

Lemon socks can be added later in the night if the child becomes hot and restless, but this treatment usually works for the first half of the night on its own, and frequently until morning.

Chapter Eight

Remedy Recipes

Elderberry Syrup

The elderberries appear after the fragrant white flowers, which are harvested for elderflower cordial and tea in the summer. The berries are a deep, dark purple and appear almost black. They can be harvested through August and into November (in the Northern Hemisphere), and must be ripe i.e. black in colour before being used for this syrup. If you are at all uncertain picking your own berries, then I would advise buying them.

There are several ways to get hold of the berries. Dried elderberries (Sambucus Nigra) can be ordered from any reputable purveyor of herbs (please see Resources section for suggestions). Fresh elderberries can be harvested from elder trees found growing wild in woodland, in hedgerows or wasteland around the British countryside. Elder trees are commonly found in people's gardens without them even realising what they are. I would suggest either finding a good book to help you identify the elder tree, Sambucus Nigra, and its berries, or find decent images on the internet so you are certain of the fruit you are picking.

Avoid eating the berries raw, as cooking enhances digestibility.

You can collect either bottles or jars, preferably ones made of dark glass and about 120-150mls in size. If you are not able to collect enough bottles, then they can be ordered off the internet from a huge number of sources. Brown or blue glass bottles are best to preserve the contents, but clear glass bottles or jars, providing they are kept away from sunlight, are fine too.

You will need:

Ingredients
- Elderberries
- Water
- Sugar, or, if your child is over one year old, you can substitute with honey

Equipment
- A measuring jug.
- Glass bottles or containers to keep the syrup in – they need to be able to be sterilized. Note that lids with rubber seals cannot be sterilised in the oven. They may need to be put through a hot wash in the dishwasher or boiled as an alternative.
- A sieve lined with either some strong kitchen towel, a clean muslin, or coffee filter paper, or
- A preserves or jelly making 'bag'. You will know what I am referring to if you have one!
- A large saucepan big enough to hold the berries you have picked and water.
- A spoon
- A potato masher (optional)

This is a very easy recipe because it is based on simple proportions. Measure the quantity of berries you have collected, for example in a measuring jug, or using pint glasses or cups. Then add half the quantity of water to the berries.

Example:
- one litre of berries
- one half litre (or 500mls) of water
  Or
- two pint glasses of berries
- one pint glass of water
  Or
- four cups of berries
- two cups of water
  You get the idea…

I use a potato masher to mash and bruise the elderberries slightly before boiling. Again, it's not necessary, but I feel it helps to release the goodness.

Bring the berries (stripped from the plant) and water in the correct proportions to the boil. Once the mixture has reached a boil, cover and allow the mixture to simmer gently for 20-30 minutes.

Pop a sieve lined with a muslin or even a sieve lined with a layer of strong kitchen towel or coffee filter paper over your measuring jug directly or over a bowl. Pour the liquid and plant material through the lined sieve slowly. Measure the liquid that has been left in the bowl or measuring jug. Whatever the quantity of liquid you have, add half the amount of sugar or honey.

Example:
- Two litres of juice
- One kg of sugar (or honey)
  Or
- Two cups of juice
- One cup of sugar (or honey)
  Or
- Two pints of juice
- One pint of sugar (or honey)
  and so on....

Return the juice to a clean saucepan. If you are using sugar then add the correct quantity of sugar to the juice in the pan now; if you are using honey, do not add this to the berry juice until it has been returned to the boil.

I find it easiest to sterilise my glass bottles or glass containers in the oven, but you may have your own way of doing it. Feel free to follow your own methods.

Heat the oven up to 130 degrees centigrade, (266 degrees Fahrenheit) and place bottles (without lids or any rubber seal bits) onto a baking tray, lying down on their sides but not touching each other. Place baking tray with bottles into the oven and "bake" for about 20 minutes. Remove the baking tray from the oven and put on the worktop on a heat-proof mat. Using oven gloves, stand the bottles up.

Return your mixture to the heat and bring it back to the boil, stirring and dissolving the sugar for a further 10 minutes. If you are using honey, then you can just stir the honey into the boiling juice and remove from the heat once the honey is well mixed in and dissolved. Honey does not need to be cooked in the same way that sugar does.

Pour the hot syrup into hot, sterilised bottles and place lids on bottles. Once the mixture has cooled you can label and date the bottles and store in a cool dark place. These should last for up to six months providing the integrity of the seal isn't compromised.

Chapter Nine

Recipes During Illness

This section contains some ideas and recipes for babies and children who are unwell and suffering acutely with a fever. You may notice that the recipes all have a high fluid content with very simple and easily digested foods — primarily fruits and herbal tea. Herbal teas contain a great deal of nutrition in the form of vital minerals and vitamins, as well as energy in the form of a sweetener, providing nourishment to a child without the need to burden their digestive system. Also, these recipes eliminate the common causes of digestive irritation such as dairy and gluten, allowing the body to focus solely on fighting infection.

Don't be alarmed if during the acute phase of illness your child has no appetite at all. Keep offering frequent, small amounts of fluids and gradually as they become well again their appetite will return. Of course, if your baby hasn't yet been weaned then breast milk, formula, cool boiled water and cool boiled herbal teas are best.

Banana Ice Cream
(Dairy free, gluten free, vegan)

Ingredients
- Four ripe bananas
- Half a cup of unsweetened plant-based milk

You Will Need
- A baking tray
- Grease proof paper, or baking parchment
- Freezer space
- A blender

Method

Peel the bananas. If you have a powerful blender such as a Vitamix, then roughly chop bananas in halves or quarters. If you have a normal blender or NutriBullet-type blender, then slice bananas into slices about one cm in thickness. Line your baking tray with the grease proof paper or baking parchment and place banana slices onto tray making sure that the slices are evenly spread out on the baking tray. Place the baking tray with banana slices into the freezer.

Once the banana slices are frozen (approximately one hour depending on how full your freezer is and how thin your banana slices are) take the slices of banana off the baking tray and put straight into the blender with your chosen plant-based milk. Whizz together in the blender until bananas are smooth and creamy. Serve immediately with whatever toppings you desire or simply plain.

Fruit Puree
(Dairy free, gluten free, vegan)

Ingredients
- Four small apples
  or
- Two to three large/medium sized apples
  or
- Four pears
- One to two tablespoons of water

You Will Need
- A vegetable peeler
- A saucepan
- A handheld blender (or potato masher if total smoothness of the puree isn't essential!)

Method

Peel the fruit and chop into quarters to remove the core. Roughly chop the fruit into small pieces, approximately one to two cm squared. Place the fruit into the saucepan along with the water and bring to the boil over a medium heat. Allow the fruit to simmer until it is very soft. Stir the fruit all the time it is simmering. Add more water if you notice the fruit sticking to the saucepan. Once the fruit is really soft, either mash it or whizz it smooth with your handheld blender. Allow the puree to cool and serve, or it can be frozen for later.

For extra nutrition or sweetness, a date can be added and simmered in with the fruit, or two dried apricots or perhaps a couple of raisins… you can experiment!

Herbal Tea Ice Lollies or Ice Cubes
(Dairy free, gluten free, vegan)

Ingredients
- Herbal tea of your choice
- 250ml or one cup of water
- Sweetener of your choice (optional)

You Will Need
- A teapot or covered vessel to brew tea in
- A kettle
- Ice lolly holders or ice cube tray

Method
Boil the kettle and brew herbal tea as if you were making a cup. Sweeten to taste and allow tea to cool. Pour tea into ice lolly moulds or ice cube tray and freeze.

Herbal Iced Tea
(Dairy free, gluten free, vegan)

Ingredients
- Herbal tea of your choice (four tea bags, or four teaspoons of loose herbs)
- 500–1000 ml (two to four cups) of freshly boiled water
- Half a fresh lemon
- Berries, fruit or vegetables of your choice! We love fresh green apple sliced small, strawberries or raspberries and peeled cucumber, but you can mix it up however you like using whatever you have. Slices of fresh orange are also great – they look lovely and help with flavour too.
- Sweetener of your choice
- Fresh herbs such as mint or basil (optional)
- Ice cubes

You Will Need
- A teapot, jug or other covered vessel to brew your tea in
- A kettle
- A large jug to mix your iced tea in

Method
Brew your tea and allow it to cool. Then add a squeeze of half a fresh lemon to your brewed herbal tea and sweeten to taste. Transfer the tea into a large jug and keep refrigerated. When your child is ready for some iced tea, choose a suitable glass. Chop up the fruits or vegetables that you are using in your tea (much like you would when mixing Pimms). Add the fruit and any fresh herbs, (if you have decided to include them), to your glass. The fruit and herbs should fill the glass somewhere between a quarter and a third full. Add a couple of ice cubes and pour cool tea over the top. Take a straw and give the mixture a stir. Serve immediately. You can go really crazy and decorate with cocktail umbrellas and flashing ice cubes – be as creative as you like!

Herbal Jelly
(Dairy free, gluten free)

Ingredients
- Herbal tea of your choice
- 250 ml or one cup of freshly boiled water
- 250 ml or one cup of pure fruit juice
- 20g of powdered or leaf gelatine
- Optional fresh fruit (such as chopped pineapple, raspberries or strawberries)

You Will Need
- A teapot, mug or other vessel to brew herbal tea in
- A kettle
- A saucepan
- A dish or container to allow the jelly to set in
- A fridge with space in!

Method
Brew the herbal tea in 250 ml of freshly boiled water. Once the herbal tea has brewed for sufficient time, remove the herbs and add the tea to the saucepan. Add 250 ml of pure fruit juice to the tea in the saucepan and prepare gelatine according to the instructions on the packet. Warm the tea and fruit juice in the saucepan, adding the gelatine, stirring all the while until the gelatine is completely dissolved. Once the gelatine is dissolved pour the mixture into the dish and allow it to cool. Once the mixture is cool the chopped fruit can be added (which is optional), before putting the mixture into the fridge for several hours to set.

Once set, the jelly is ready to serve and enjoy.

Spiced Mylk
(Dairy free, gluten free, vegan)

Ingredients
- 500 ml or two cups of dairy free milk, such as almond, Koko (derived from coconut), oat milk, rice milk, soya milk, whatever your preference. Of course, you can always use cows' milk if you prefer. In our family, we love this made with cashew nut milk.
- One to two teaspoons of honey or other sweetener of your choice
- Three cardamom pods that have been bashed and bruised either in a pestle and mortar or with a large knife handle, rolling pin, end of a wine bottle, you get what I mean!
- One teaspoon of ground cinnamon, or about two inches of cinnamon stick
- One teaspoon of ground turmeric
- Three black pepper corns, or a dash of freshly ground pepper

You Will Need
- A saucepan
- A whisk
- A mug or cup
- A pestle and mortar or other implement to bash cardamom pods
- A tea strainer or sieve

Method
Bash up the cardamom pods so that they are open and bruised. Put them in the saucepan, seeds and all. Pour milk into the saucepan and add all the other ingredients. Whisk them all together whilst gently warming the milk on the stove top. When the milk nears boiling point or you see it start to bubble, turn off the heat and cover the pan, allowing the mixture to infuse for 10 minutes. Once it has infused, whisk the milk to ensure all the ingredients are well combined and pour into a mug through a tea strainer or sieve to ensure all seeds, pods, sticks and peppercorns are removed. Taste and sweeten further if necessary. Allow to cool so it is still warm, yet cool enough to serve and drink.

Broth
(Dairy free, vegan)

This is an excellent way to replenish important salts and nutrients in a child who may be dehydrated or who has sweated a lot with a fever. It is also a useful fluid to give during diarrhoea and/or once any vomiting has subsided.

Ingredients
- One half to one full teaspoon of Marigold Organic Swiss, Reduced Salt, Vegetable Bouillon (Vegan Bouillon is also an option)
- 250 ml (one cup) freshly boiled water

You Will Need
- A teaspoon
- A kettle
- A mug or jug

Method
Boil 250 ml of fresh water and pour into a mug or jug. Add anything from a half a teaspoon to a whole teaspoon of bouillon, depending on the age and taste of your child. Stir the bouillon until it has thoroughly mixed and dissolved in the hot water. Allow the mixture to cool until it is just warmer than body temperature and give to the child in small sips.

Fruit Kanten
(Dairy free, gluten free, vegan)

This is like a jelly but made with a gelatine-type substance derived from seaweed. As such, it contains wonderful minerals and nutrients, but is without colour, flavour or taste. Perfect for children!

Ingredients
- One cup of thinly sliced fruit (my favourites are strawberries, peaches, nectarines or grapes)
- 500 ml (two cups) of apple juice
- Two tablespoons of Agar-Agar flakes (available in most Health Food shops and good supermarkets in the Oriental Foods section)

You Will Need
- A saucepan
- A dish
- Fridge space

Method
Place your sliced fruit in your dish. Pour the apple juice into the saucepan and bring to a gentle boil. Stir in the Agar-Agar until it is dissolved, which can take five minutes or more. Once it has thoroughly dissolved pour the mixture over your fruit in the bowl and allow it to cool. Once cool place the mixture in the fridge for two hours, or until it has set. Then it's ready to serve.

Chapter Ten

Recipes for Recovery

This section offers some suggestions for providing nutrition and fluids to a child who is recovering from being unwell. You may notice that many of the recipes are high in calories and also nutritionally dense, with food in its softest and most easily absorbed form. These are the general principles to follow when your child's appetite returns after a fever. However, you may have your own recipes and family traditions surrounding food and illness, and generally your child will be very clear about what foods they feel like eating. I tend to go with the cravings my children have because it shows that they are listening to their body and this is something I want to encourage.

Of course, these recipes are only appropriate for babies who are already weaned, until then breast milk or formula is best.

Strawberry Cream
(Dairy free, gluten free, vegan)

Ingredients
- 260g strawberries de-stemmed
- Three ripe bananas, chopped and frozen beforehand
- A couple of drops of vanilla extract or seeds scraped from half a vanilla pod (optional

You Will Need
- A blender
- Glasses or bowl to serve in
- Spoons to eat it with! Or maybe a straw to suck it up, depending on your mood and the thickness of the cream.

Method
Place all the ingredients together in a blender and whizz until the ingredients are thick and creamy in consistency. Serve immediately. If you would like a sweeter cream, then a date or two can be added to all the ingredients in the blender and whizzed up.

Overnight Egg Custard
(Gluten free)

Ingredients
- One whole egg per person
- 160 ml full fat milk per egg
- One tablespoon of sugar (white or brown) or coconut sugar
- One quarter teaspoon of vanilla extract per egg

You Will Need
- An egg poacher pan
  Or
- Small, clean glass jars with lids (think jam jars), which can fit in a saucepan with the saucepan lid on
  Or
- Ramekin-type dish covered with tin foil and secured with an elastic band around the top of each ramekin
- A saucepan
- Water

Method
Collect as many egg-poaching pan containers or jars or ramekins as the number of eggs you are using. For example, five eggs=five people=five jars, ramekins or egg poaching pan containers. Mix all the ingredients together until the mixture is thick and frothy and then divide the mixture evenly between your chosen containers. Secure lids to jars or foil over ramekins. Place jars or ramekins into a saucepan and fill the saucepan with water so that the water in the saucepan is approximately the same height as the egg mixture in the containers. If you are using an egg-poaching pan, fill the pan with water and place the egg-poaching dishes in their slots. Cover the egg-poaching pan with its lid. Bring the water to the boil.

Once the water is boiling turn off the heat and keep the lid on the egg-poaching pan. If you are using a saucepan, also keep the lid on. Leave like this overnight or for eight hours, after which the custard will be set. A little sprinkle of nutmeg can be grated over the top of each serving if desired.

Simple Rice Pudding

Ingredients
- One cup of already cooked rice (this is a great recipe for leftover rice!) Basmati rice works well with this, but any type of cooked rice will do.
- One egg, beaten
- Three tablespoons of honey, or other sweetener of your choice
- A small handful of currants, raisins and/or chopped almonds
- Full fat milk or cream

You Will Need
- A saucepan

Method
Gently mix the rice, beaten egg, honey and currents, raisins and/or chopped almonds in the saucepan. Mix slowly and carefully so that the rice doesn't go all mushy. Pour in enough milk or cream so that it is equal with the level of the top of the rice mixture, so barely covering the rice. Cook over a low heat for five to eight minutes, stirring slowly so that the rice doesn't turn to porridge. Serve immediately.

Vegan Rice Pudding
(Dairy free, vegan)

Ingredients
- One x 400ml tin of coconut milk
- 200g of pudding or short-grain rice
- 400ml unsweetened almond or soya milk
- Three tablespoons of honey or other sweetener of your choice
- Two teaspoons of vanilla extract or seeds scraped from one vanilla pod
- One tablespoon of coconut oil
- Jam (optional, as garnish!)

You Will Need
- A saucepan

Method
Add the coconut milk, rice, almond or soya milk and the honey or sweetener of your choice to the pan. Stir while slowly bringing the mixture to a gentle simmer. Add the vanilla and stir it into the mixture, cover the pan with a lid and allow to very gently simmer for 20-25 minutes, checking and giving the rice a stir frequently. Taste the rice after this time to make sure that it is thoroughly soft and cooked.

Turn the heat off, stir in the tablespoon of coconut oil and cover the pan once more with the lid and leave for 10 minutes. If necessary, you can thin the pudding slightly by adding a small amount of warm water or warm almond milk. Serve into bowls and add a spoonful of jam to the centre of each serving of rice pudding, just like they used to at school if you fancy a flashback to the good old days.

Rice Porridge

I lived overseas for much of my childhood, often in countries where diarrhoea and sickness were common. A doctor in the Philippines first prescribed rice porridge for me when I was very young and unwell. It is nourishing, strengthening and very easily absorbed and processed by the body. It consists of salts, sugars, fluids, carbohydrates, vitamins and minerals; ideal for rehydrating and replenishing a child. I have included a basic recipe, as well as a more involved recipe which is more nutritionally dense and will really help to restore health and vitality to a child who has been unwell.

Basic Recipe

Ingredients
- One litre of freshly boiled water
- Quarter cup of white rice, (preferably basmati). This can be changed to brown rice if the child has had no gastrointestinal disturbance such as diarrhoea
- Four teaspoons of Marigold Organic Swiss, Reduced Salt, Vegetable Bouillon

You Will Need
- A large saucepan

Method

Put the the rice in the saucepan, add the freshly boiled litre of water and the four teaspoons of bouillon and stir. Put the pan on the heat and bring to the boil. Remove any scum that rises to the top with a spoon. Reduce the heat and simmer, stirring occasionally, for about 40 minutes if it's white rice and an hour if it's brown rice. Take off the heat, ladle into bowls and serve.

Alternative Recipe

Ingredients
- One litre of fresh chicken stock
- Quarter cup of white rice, (preferably basmati). This can be changed to brown rice if the child has had no gastrointestinal disturbance such as diarrhoea

- One carrot, peeled and chopped very finely
- One stick of celery, chopped very finely
- A sprinkle of fresh parsley to garnish (optional, but nutritionally very beneficial!)

You Will Need
- A large saucepan

Method

Put the rice in the saucepan and add the litre of fresh chicken stock. Put the pan on the heat and bring to the boil. Remove any scum that rises to the top with a spoon. Reduce the heat and simmer, stirring occasionally, for about 40 minutes if it's white rice and an hour if it's brown rice. Add the finely chopped vegetables to the porridge and allow to simmer for a further 15 minutes or until they are soft and tender. Season with sea salt if necessary, then serve in bowls with a garnish of fresh parsley sprinkled over the top.

You can increase the nutritional and restorative value of this porridge exponentially by adding small pieces of cooked chicken, a pinch of turmeric or other vegetables, and even a beaten egg.

Egg Soup

Ingredients
- 125-250ml freshly boiled water
- One organic, free range fresh egg yolk per 125ml water
- one half to one teaspoon of Marigold Organic Swiss, Reduced Salt, Vegetable Bouillon
- A sprinkling of fresh parsley to garnish (optional)

You Will Need
- A saucepan

Method
Pour the freshly boiled water into the saucepan and bring to a rolling boil. To the water add either half a teaspoon of bouillon to 125ml of water, or the full teaspoon of bouillon if you have used 250ml of water. In the meantime, separate the egg white from the yolk and set aside. Pour the boiled bouillon into either a bowl or mug and add the egg yolk to the bouillon whole.

Allow the egg yolk to sit whole in the soup for five minutes so it can cook before serving. The egg yolk will be runny and can be broken once in the soup and mixed in giving the soup a delicious taste, a thicker texture and your child some good nutrition. Kids usually like to be the ones to break it with their spoon and mix it in themselves!

Simple Chicken Broth/Stock

Ingredients
- Chicken bones – usually two to three carcasses from a roast chicken dinner. Just stick the chicken carcass in the freezer when you have used all the meat and it will keep until you are ready or need to make some stock.
- Chicken feet (optional, but it does provide extra nutrition and gelatine. They are usually available from your local butcher.)
- One onion chopped into quarters
- One carrot chopped into quarters
- Two tablespoons of vinegar
- Cold water to cover the bones

You Will Need
- A slow cooker
  Or
- A large saucepan
- Tongs or a slotted spoon
- A bowl or container (large enough to hold approximately two litres of stock)

Method
Place the chicken bones, feet, onion and carrot in either a large pan or slow cooker. Add the vinegar and fill the pan or slow cooker with enough cold water to just cover the bones. Let this stand for at least half an hour to 45 minutes to allow the vinegar to start softening the chicken bones and enable the minerals and goodness to be released from them. If using a slow cooker, cook on a low heat for 8-12 hours, checking periodically to ensure that water is just covering the bones at all times, and adding more when necessary. If cooking on a stove-top, bring the liquid to the boil and reduce the heat to a rolling, gentle simmer for 6-8 hours, and please don't leave it unattended in the house. Always make sure there is enough water covering the bones by checking regularly.

When this is complete, turn the heat off and remove bones and vegetables with tongs and/or slotted spoon. They can all be added to the compost.

Strain the stock through a fine mesh strainer into a jug, bowl or other heatproof container. The stock can be used straight away, but it can also be allowed to cool and then either refrigerated or frozen. It can keep in the fridge for up to five days and for much longer (several months) in the freezer.

Once the stock is cool and has set, the congealed fat can be scraped off the top of the stock and discarded if you prefer.

Resources

These are mainly UK based resources (apart from the books). A short search online in whichever country you live should quickly reveal relevant organisations and distributers closer to you. This is simply a small list of suggestions for products I have found useful and effective and have used regularly – I would love to hear about any you have tried and loved!

Books

Aromatherapy

Aromatherapy for the Healthy Child (2000) Valerie Ann Worwood; New World Library, California

The Complete Book of Essential Oils and Aromatherapy (1990) Valerie Ann Worwood; Macmillan, London

The Directory of Essential Oils (2001) Wanda Sellar; C.W. Daniel Company Ltd.

Conventional Medicine

How to Raise a Healthy Child... In Spite of Your Doctor (1987) Robert S. Mendelsohn M.D.; The Random House Publishing Group, Toronto

Real Medicine, Real Health (2004) Dr. Arden Anderson; Holographic Health Press, Waynesville, N.C.

The Vaccine-Friendly Plan, Dr. Paul's Safe and Effective Approach to Immunity and Health – From Pregnancy Through Your Child's Teen Years (2016) Paul Thomas M.D. and Jennifer Margulis Ph.D.; Ballantine Books, New York

Cook Books

Boost Your Child's Immune System (2010) Lucy Burney; Piatkus Books, London

Optimum Nutrition for Babies and Young Children, Over 150 Quick and Tempting Recipes For The Best Start in Life (2010) Lucy Burney; Piatkus Books, London

River Cottage Baby and Toddler Cookbook (2011) Nikki Duffy; Bloomsbury Publishing PLC, London

The Mystic Cookfire, The Sacred Art of Creating Food to Nurture Friends and Family (2011) Veronika Sophia Robinson; Starflower Press

Herbs

Green Pharmacy, The History and Evolution of Western Herbal Medicine (1997) Barbara Griggs; Healing Arts Press, Vermont

Hedgerow Medicine (2008) Julie Bruton-Seal, Matthew Seal; Merlin Unwin

Herbal Healers – 21 Familiar Kitchen and Garden Herbs (1999) Glennie Kindred; Wooden Books

Herbal Medicine (1993) Dian Dincin Buchman; Tiger Books International PLC, Twickenham

Herbal Remedies for Children's Health (1999) Rosemary Gladstar; Storey Publishing, USA

Letting in the Wild Edges (2013) Glennie Kindred; Permanent Publications, UK

The Herbal for Mather & Child (2003) Anne McIntyre; Throsons, London

Wise Woman Herbal for the Childbearing Year (1986) Susun S. Weed; Ashtree Publishing, Woodstock, New York

Homeopathy

Homeopathic Medicine for Children and Infants (1992) Dana Ullman; Penguin Putnam Inc. New York

The Family Guide to Homeopathy (1989) Dr Andrew Lockie; Guild Publishing, London

The Science of Homeopathy (1988) George Vithoulkas; Grove Press Inc. New York

Apothecaries, Pharmacies and Suppliers of Medicines

Aromatherapy

Neal's Yard www.nealsyardremedies.com
Quinessence www.quinessence.co.uk

Flower Remedies

Healing Herbs Bach Flower Essences www.healingherbs.co.uk
Dr. Hauschka www.dr.hauschka.com

Herbs

Botanica Medica www.botanicamedica.co.uk
Urban Fringe, Bristol www.urbanfringe.co.uk

Homeopathy

Ainsworths www.ainsworths.com
Helios www.helios.co.uk
Weleda www.weleda.co.uk

Useful Websites, Organisations and Phone Numbers

Arnica Uk Parents' Support Network www.arnica.org.uk
The Aromatherapy Council UK www.aromatherapycouncil.org.uk
Homeopathy Helpline 0906 534 3404 (Premium call rate, UK only) or
    for worldwide access to advice visit www.homeopathyhelpline.com to
    arrange skype or email consultation.
NHS Helpline 111 (UK only, free to call)
National Institute for Care Excellence (NICE) www.nice.org.uk

General Osteopathic Council www.osteopathy.org.uk
The National Institute of Medical Herbalists www.nmih.org.uk
The Society of Homeopaths www.homeopathy-soh.org

Aromatherapy Vaporisers and Diffusers

Aroma-Stone www.nealsyardremedies.com and www.amazon.co.uk
Aroma-Stream www.amazon.co.uk
Aroma Diffuser by Stadler Form (my current favourite!)
www.stadlerform.com and www.amazon.co.uk

Baby Weaning Cups

www.babycup.co.uk

Bambino Merino Sleeping Bags

www.naturalbabyshower.co.uk

Herbal Teas

Hambledon Herbs www.hambledenherbs.com
Floradix www.amazon.co.uk
Organic India www.organicindia.co.uk
Yogi Tea www.yogitea.com
Dr. Stuart's www.drstuarts.com
Sidroga www.amazon.uk unless you have friends and family in mainland Europe

Herbal Syrups

Elderberry
Dol Rosa Canina www.dolrosacanina.co.uk
Pukka Elderberry Syrup www.pukkaherbs.com
Biona Elderberry Juice www.biona.co.uk

Lime Flower
Dol Rosa Canina www.dolrosacanina.co.uk

Himalayan Salt Lamps

The largest variety I have found is on www.amazon.co.uk

Munchkin Fresh Food Feeder

www.munchkin.com

Oral Syringes and Droppers
The largest variety I found on www.amazon.co.uk

Suppliers of Dark Glass Bottles
www.baldwins.co.uk amongst many many others!

NOTES

NOTES

NOTES

NOTES

NOTES

NOTES

NOTES

NOTES